CW00521651

INTENTIONAL HEALING

FROM SCARS TO STARS

STORIES OF STRENGTH, COURAGE, RESILIENCE, AND TRIUMPHANT NAVIGATION THROUGH PAIN TO HOPE AND FORGIVENESS

STORIES COMPILED BY
DR. GRACE A. KELLY

Copyright © 2022 by Dr. Grace A. Kelly
ISBN 978-976-96979-1-1 (Paperback)
Produced, Published, and Owned by Dr. Grace A. Kelly,
of The Olive Branch Global LLC
All rights reserved. No part of this publication may be reproduced, distributed, or transmitted in any form or by any means, including photography, recording, etc. without the written permission of the publisher. Limitation of Liability: Under no circumstances shall The Olive Branch Global LLC, its affiliates, or authors be liable for any indirect, incidental, consequential, special, or exemplary damages arising out of or in connection with your use of any exercises or information contained in this book. Please be advised that if you choose to follow any of the suggestions offered by the authors, you do so of your own accord.
Although this book speaks to the challenges of our contributing authors, including but not limited to abuse, grief, violence, etc., it is not designed to be a definitive guide or to take the place of a qualified professional.
For more information, please contact us at
www.theolivebranchglobal.com

This book was presented to:

. . . .

by

. . . .

on this

. . . . day of . . . .

in the year of our Lord

. . . .

ACKNOWLEDGMENT

Intentional Healing: From Scars to Stars Anthology is a God-given project and God-directed process. I want to first acknowledge and give thanks to my mentor, friend, and companion who chose me before I was born, prepared me for service, and gave me the mandate to "go tell." Mark 5:19 (KJV) says, "Go home to your friends, and tell them how great things the Lord hath done for thee and hath had compassion on thee." Allow me to acknowledge all who embraced the vision and supported the process as I remained trustworthy and true to my promises, to support thirty persons to write and publish their stories and become bestselling authors in 90 to 120 days.

Let me acknowledge my colleagues, family, and friends, especially those who stood by me during the process. To my speaking coach and #1 motivational speaker, Les Brown, for his mentorship while I was in his prodigy and speaking programmes. I remember being called out by him several times to own my God-given skills and calling. To Jessica T. Moore, my coach who stopped at nothing to ensure that I advanced from writing a chapter in an anthology to leading this anthology. Through her encouragement and motivation, I was inspired to successfully lead this anthology.

I am indebted to each co-author for accepting the challenge to own and share their truth, for going through the rigors of identifying their pain, reframing their narrative, and seeking healing for l their scars with intentionality. They are now able to retell and not relive their story while navigating their scars to shine as stars and illuminate the path for those with similar scars. Do accept the commendation and recognition you so deserve Joy Allen, Dr. Paulene Gayle-Betten, Debbie-Ann Dyer, Melva Slythe-Farquharson, Wendy Ann Forbes, Andrea Francis, Claudia V. Francia, Sashoi M. Grant, Donette A. James-Samuel, Dr. Joan M. Latty, Dr. Judith McGhie, Carmen Mahlum, Evadne McLilley, Tishauna Mullings, Raymond Nelson, Elaine Oxamendi Vicet, Latoya Pinnock-Wilson, Chauna-Kaye Pottinger, Roy Pusey, Dawn Richards, Dawn 'Lady

D' Samuels, Stacia Samuels, Dr. Ivanah Thomas, Jackie Thaw, Dr. Keisha Ann Thomas, La-Toya Arthur-Tucker, Jodine Joanna Williams, Joyce V. Williams, and Dr. Patrice Wright.

Family is one of the strongest and most essential support systems ordained by God. I acknowledge and say thank you to all my family members who believed in me, validated my effort, and embraced my vision for this anthology and my life work as a grief and bereavement therapist coach. Of special mention are my siblings Eulin (Annette), Doreen (Aunty Gaye), Errol (Lenkey/Harper), and Mama's "wash belly" Arnold (Chummy). Thanks for your love and support.

For moral, technical, and other support, La-Toya Arthur, Jodine Williams, Arif Hossain, Janet Livingston, Princess Lawes, and Ryan McCalla. Finally, I wish to acknowledge you, yes you, who have chosen to purchase, read this book, and take the necessary steps towards intentional healing. As you navigate your scars, name them, separate them from yourself, disempower them, and embrace the stars within you.

DEDICATION

This anthology is firstly dedicated to God who gave the mandate, inspired the vision, and guided and empowered the visionary authors in using this medium to share stories of strength, courage, resilience, triumph through pain, and hope, and forgiveness. All praise and honour to God for creating this community of visionary game-changers.

To Urina Taylor Kelly, mother of Dr. Grace A. Kelly, whose death caused the excruciating pain that has fuelled Dr. Kelly's passion to be a subject matter expert and trailblazer in providing effective grief coaching services to many across the globe. Thanks also to President Lincoln Ewards, Vice President Vivienne Quarrie, and Mrs. Aalia Muatafaa Wiliams for the professional courtesies extended.

We also dedicate this work to significant persons in the life of the co-authors.

Jennifer Angela Brown
Dr. Duane Covrig
Utah Dunstan-Phillips
Beverly Adella Francis
Errol James Francis
Isolyn Gracey Harris
Edna Graver-Scringer
Jediel Jenae Tucker
Vivian Jones
Joseph Latty
Munganyinka Liberathe
Claudette Myers
Florence Pearlene "Normsie" Nelson
Joanne Palmer
Veeveet Kelly Peterkin
Kathleen Pusey
Jean Richards
Viris Victoria Reddie
Dr. Beverly Rose
Lenworth Rose
Josiah Samuel Wilson
Patrick Thaw
Inez Thompson
Rose Williams
Roy Williams
Verona Williams
Jazmyne Williams

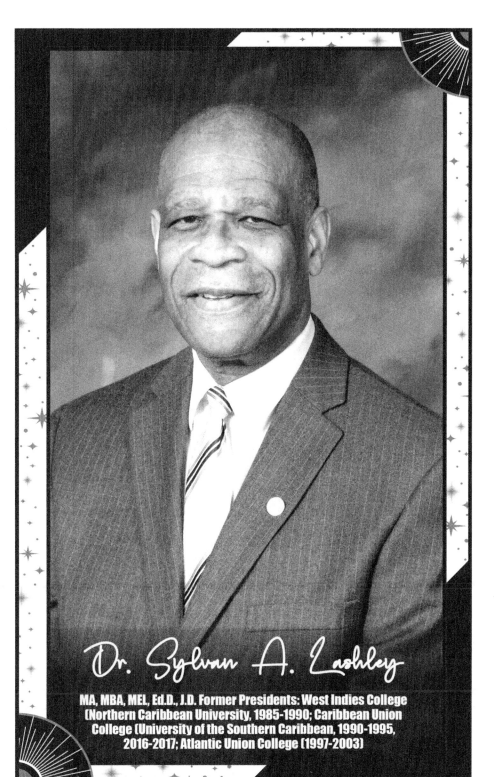

Dr. Sylvan A. Lashley

MA, MBA, MEL, Ed.D., J.D. Former Presidents: West Indies College
(Northern Caribbean University, 1985-1990; Caribbean Union
College (University of the Southern Caribbean, 1990-1995,
2016-2017; Atlantic Union College (1997-2003)

Foreword
"FROM SCARS TO STARS"

It gives me great pleasure to write the foreword to this remarkable Anthology. I was privileged to find and recruit the author when she was a young teen in Montego Bay, Jamaica, and I invited her to the then West Indies College (now Northern Caribbean University) in Mandeville, Jamaica, where I served as president. I remember that eventful day as I drove by, slowed down, and wondered whether to stop, as I spied "the young girl" perched under a mango tree. So, I stopped, introduced myself, and she came to campus to take up her first job in the ladies residence (Jamaica Hall), that of maintaining the lobby floors as a work-scholarship, for there was no money. An astounding summer job of glittery and glimmering floors was followed by further work assignments and scholarships to take her through the year. There was little money, but tremendous will on her part. She went through the scars of the beginning, to the stars of the completing, from struggle to triumph and to victory. She inspired all and repeated the process. I became the president of two other Adventist colleges, became a dean of continuing education, dean of a School of Business, and completed my further graduate degrees spurred on by the faith and fortitude of a memory of this author. This student quietly became the teacher in a complete role reversal. Each of us, therefore, is a teacher in his/her own right, for in teaching and learning, professor and student represent one continuous art form in the synchronous and asynchronous space.

Dr. Grace A. Kelly is the best person to lead this Anthology, Intentional Healing: From Scars to Stars, because she visibly and audibly represents the lived experiences of the persons she describes—she has trod that path before and has taken "the road hardly travelled." She has drunk from the bitter bottom of the cup to the sweet flavorings at the top, but sometimes, the bitter comes before the sweet as better comes before best. She serves at the Northern Caribbean University in the areas of counseling and education. She extends her expertise in the areas of crisis intervention, grief, and bereavement therapy. She has also served as a lay preacher, a Red Cross Psycho-social First Aid Responder and Trainer, and President of the Jamaica Association of Guidance Counsellors in Education. Dr. Grace writes from a background of practical experience, rather than mere theoretical research. She demonstrates and describes the sequence of the human psycho-social life-span, through the Anthology and in her own life, reminding us that while we encounter the scars of a desert experience, the stars of an oasis await us. This journey has led her into restorative justice and training as a way to heal the scars of serious offenses, signaling that there is always mercy and grace.

This Anthology serves as a catalyst for healing, personal reflection, and professional development. Although challenged by the grief and crisis of the COVID-19 pandemic, the Anthology offers an opportunity for psycho-social study and reflection. The Anthology, which is an international perspective of a psycho-social compass due to its diversity of contributors, reminds of Erik Erikson's eight-stage theory of psycho-social development (Cherry, 2022) of trust vs. mistrust (infancy from birth to 18 months), autonomy vs. shame and doubt (the toddler years from 18 months to three years), initiative vs. inferiority (the middle school years of six to eleven), identity vs. confusion (the young adult years from eighteen to of forty), generativity vs. stagnation (the years from the middle ages of 40 to 65), and the final stage of integrity vs. despair (the older adulthood from 65 to death).

The international collection of stories makes the book a universal treasure and comes on the heels of her first book Grieve If You Must: a 21-day Plan for Grieving, Healing and Restoration. We must all encounter the desert and make an effort to reach the oases. I heartily recommend this book of healing to the readership as a life-changing event. Scars can turn to stars as the desert becomes an oasis, for without scars, there will be little appreciation for the stars. It is not the scars that count, but the stars that matter. By beholding the North Star, the South Scar seems to matter little in our quest and journey to complete freedom and absolution from grief and despair. So, young men and young women, find your North Star and forget the South Scar. Go quickly now, run, and do not be weary. Read slowly and surely.

Sincerely,

Sylvan A. Lashley

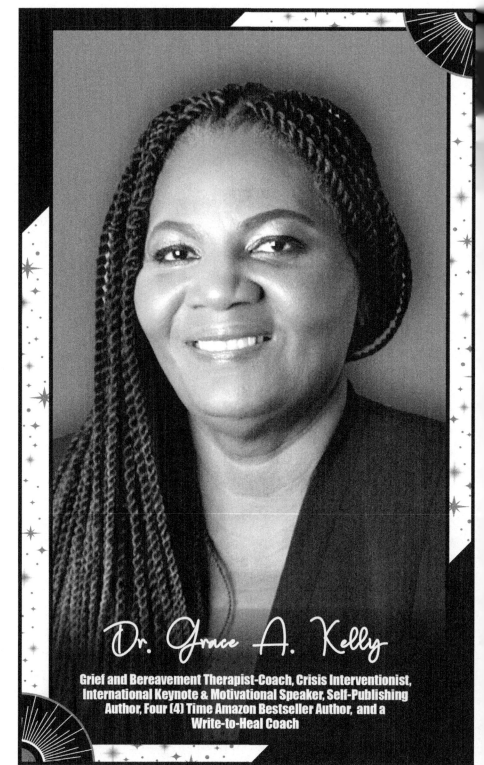

Dr. Grace A. Kelly

Grief and Bereavement Therapist-Coach, Crisis Interventionist, International Keynote & Motivational Speaker, Self-Publishing Author, Four (4) Time Amazon Bestseller Author, and a Write-to-Heal Coach

PREFACE

"There is no grief like the grief that does not speak."
-Henry Wadsworth Longfellow

In 2007, after a series of deaths, including my sister Olive on October 1, I knew I had to do something. Identifying what to do was as difficult as finding a specific grain of sand in the ocean span across the world. At that time, I had been, and perhaps was still teaching Techniques of Counselling at both the graduate and undergraduate levels. The undergraduate text was Intentional Interviewing and Counseling, 5th edition, 2003 by E. Allen and Mary Bradford Ivey. They defined intentionality as acting with a sense of capability and deciding from among a range of alternative actions. They further stated that the intentional individual has more than one action, thought, or behavior from which to choose in responding to changing life situations, being able to generate alternatives in a given situation and approach a problem from different vantage points, using a variety of skills and personal attributes. I was fascinated by the concept of embracing it and found it to be very useful in my class activities and counselling practice.

Naturally, when I was in the darkest hours of my grief and did not know if there was a way out, I decided to try something new. I became intentional about healing my scars. My identified scars covered me like an intricately designed full-body tattoo with associated emotions that enveloped me like a tightly folded cabbage. I remember thinking, Who on earth can help me? No one responded and the sound of my unspoken words echoed into nothingness. Then the inspiration to assign myself as my client, as I would normally pair my technique students to treat each other's presenting problems, engulfed me. Their presenting problems could have been made-up but mine were real. They were two, and it was only me. One. The pain left me thinking, do or die. The desire to do was pursued. Hence, I am here interacting with you.

I proceeded in scheduling times to grieve and designed a 21-day treatment plan for myself. I applied my three-stage formula for grieving, healing, and restoration, using the skills, techniques, and the recommended guide by Ivey and Ivey (2002). To encourage me along the journey, I practiced micro shifts and positive habit stocking as I got better at managing my grief. That process became my guide and led me to a healthier and more fulfilling way of life. The benefits were rewarding. This was validated by the impact my story had on a young woman who inadvertently bumped into it on my desk at home and started reading.

I found her sobbing as though she had gotten death news–but somehow with a look of relief. After enquiring what happened, she said something to this effect, "You don't know Miss Grace, you don't know." As I looked at my script in her hand, without hesitation, she shared how reading my story helped her come to grips with something with which she had been struggling for years. I shared what happened with my friend and colleague Dr. Pearnell Bell, who is a Clinical Psychologist. She read my story and agreed that it was a powerful tool that could help others and encouraged me to complete the process. The manuscript was revised to produce a book, which as a reviewer, she commented, "Dr. Kelly's book Grieve If You Must, gives the mourner permission to grieve and guides them with grace and ease through what is a very difficult period." Wendel Abel, MPh, DM, Consultant Psychiatrist & Head, Section of Psychiatry, Dept. of Community Health and Psychiatry, University of the West Indies, who penned the foreword of the book said, "This book represents an attempt to bring the opportunity of healing to the conflict of grief. It further furnishes individuals with a great opportunity for the understanding of the grief and healing processes, while providing great insight into their condition, which helps them work through their emotions." Sandra Eleanor McDermott, PsyD, LLP, CCFC – Clinical Psychologist, in the preface of the said book declared, "The book is fairly balanced and easy to read and understand. Provisions are made by the author for the reader to complete experiential assignments in order to resolve intra-psychic tension stemming from unresolved grief." Other reviews and greater details of how this process works can be found in my first book, titled Grieve If You Must: A 21-day Plan for Grieving, Healing and Restoration, now available at AdventSource and soon to be on Amazon.

Recognizing how, after those scars I bore were healed, I became more compassionate, committed, and passionate about supporting and empowering people who were knocked down and scarred. The book became my guide in teaching and presenting on related topics of grief management, across the Caribbean, North, Central and South Americas, and Europe. The deep emotional response of participants' appreciation for the healing and relief experienced from interaction with the written and spoken contents of the book transcends age, sex, status, or circumstances, surrounding their pain. As a primary reference also for my radio program aired on NCU FM, A Moment With Dr. Grace, between the years 2014-2019, a YouTube feature Let's Talk Life and Legacy: A Moment With Dr. Grace aired on the Facebook page bearing the same title and my YouTube Channel Facing Life, since December 2020. This was a direct response to issues of the COVID-19 pandemic and a way to reach more persons in keeping up with the demand for my services.

The title of this anthology Intentional Healing: From Scars To Stars emerged from a later podcast that began on Clubhouse in 2021. Simultaneously, a series of presentations ended in May 2022 with individuals at the Redemption Praise Temple, where I facilitated a weekly series using the Grieve If You Must book as a guide. The results were astonishing! Reviews can be seen on the RPTTV YouTube page. Additionally, in March of 2022, I published my story entitled "From Scars to Stars" in the Jessica T. Moore bestseller Embracing Imperfections Vol. 2. This marked the beginning of the transition from a story to a book. Intentional Healing: From Scars to Stars was inspired by my knowledge and use of this approach and also the need to add unique methods for persons experiencing grief to be empowered, heal intentionally, and be liberated. Our unique methodology is the application of the principles of narrative therapy with the use of my grief concentric circle which allows authors to unpack their scars and be able to navigate them and heal one scar at a time.

As you turn the pages of this book you will find stories of strength, courage, resilience, and triumph through pain to hope, and forgiveness. Having successfully healed from those scars, I was empowered and healthily positioned to impact others. To this end, this book presents some steps for readers to intentionally navigate scars and transition from shame to self-compassion. In spite of your current or past circumstances, this book provides suggestions on how you can now reflect on the experiences of these authors and start operating out of a larger vision of yourself, knowing that you are not alone.

"When life knocks you down, try to land on your back. Because if you can look up, you can get up" (Brown, 1980). This has also become one of my favorite quotations. I often share this with individuals challenged by life circumstances. As a renowned, notable grief and bereavement therapist coach, traversing the globe, physically and virtually, I have come to realize that too often, when faced with challenges, we allow this thing called life to knock us down. My countless encounters with disappointments, obstacles, and setbacks have taught me that being knocked down is never the challenge. The true challenge is finding the courage to get back up. Even if we do get up, we are left with emotional scars that some choose to wear as a badge of honour, a symbol of shame, or victory.

You might have experienced a myriad of disappointments. Maybe you have already given up and perhaps you just need a little fire and a little encouragement to get back on your feet. This anthology opens your vision to recognize that there is a level of healing that you can achieve by writing and sharing your story. The encouragement or coaching, and insights into a different strategy or plan of action that you need may be between these pages.

To give our readers a glimpse into the Narrative Therapy concept, you will find Dr. Pearnell Bell's chapter toward the end of the book titled Healing With Intention. Additionally, information and the process of utilizing the Grief Concentric Circle can be found in Chapter 2, on pages 52-59 of the book Grieve If You Must-A 21-day Plan for Grieving Healing and Restoration.

Visionary Author,

Dr. Grace A. Kelly

TABLE OF CONTENTS

INTRODUCTION 1

CHAPTER 1: IT IS NOT THE END, IT IS ONLY A bEND 5
By: LA-TOYA ARTHUR-TUCKER

CHAPTER 2: GOD@WORK 14
By: JODINE JOANNA WILLIAMS

CHAPTER 3: KEVVIN'S SMILES: A PROMISE OF HOPE 23
By: JACQULINE THAW

CHAPTER 4: BREAKING THE SILENCE BEHIND HER GLASS DOOR 33
By: STACIA SAMUELS

CHAPTER 5: METAMORPHOSIS: MY JOURNEY TO BECOMING 42
By: DAWN RICHARDS

CHAPTER 6: KEPT 51
By: DONETTE JAMES-SAMUEL

CHAPTER 7: OUTRUNNING GRIEF 60
By: CARMEN REDDIE MAHLUM

CHAPTER 8: YOUR DREAMS MOBILIZER: THE SECRET TO GETTING 70
MORE LIVING OUT OF LIFE
By: MELVA FARQUHARSON

CHAPTER 9: ANTIFRAGILITY: GOING BEYOND RESILIENCE 79
By: TISHAUNA MULLINGS

CHAPTER 10: CIRCLE OF HOPE: JOSIAH SPEAKS HOPE 88
By: LATOYA PINNOCK-WILSON

CHAPTER 11: LOSS OF A PEARL: RECLAIMING HOPE 97
By: DR. JOAN M. LATTY

CHAPTER 12: UNDYING LOVE 106
By: DR. JUDITH MCGHIE

CHAPTER 13: A LIVING LEGACY 115
By: ANDREA FRANCIS

CHAPTER 14: REALIGNED ALLEGIANCE: TO GOD BE THE GLORY 124
By: CHAUNA-KAYE POTTINGER

CHAPTER 15: LOVING ENOUGH TO LET GO! 133
By: JOY ALLEN

CHAPTER 16: STANDING STRONG THROUGH ALONE: VOICE OF A 141
LONE SURVIVOR
By: DR. PAULENE GAYLE-BETTEN

CHAPTER 17: THE GRIEF NAVIGATOR 150
By: DR. GRACE A. KELLY

TABLE OF CONTENTS

CHAPTER 18: **PARALYZED TO BE ACTUALIZED**   158
By: Dr. Ivanah Thomas

CHAPTER 19: **OVERCOMING FEAR**   167
By: Debbie-Ann Dyer

CHAPTER 20 **UNPACKING SHAME...IMPACTING LIVES**   176
By: Elaine Oxamendi Vicet

CHAPTER 21: **UNWANTED! AUNTIED! UNDAUNTED!**   185
By: Raymond Nelson

CHAPTER 22: **FROM BROKEN-NESS TO WHOLESOME-NESS**   194
By: Dawn 'Lady D' Samuels

CHAPTER 23: **DUNCE ROW TO HONOR ROLL**   203
By: Evadne A. McLilley

CHAPTER 24: **POVERTY TO PROSPERITY: A SINGLE MOTHER'S JOURNEY**   212
By: Joyce V. Williams

CHAPTER 25: **GROWING THROUGH THE ROCKS**   221
By: Dr. Patrice Wright

CHAPTER 26: **BROKEN, BUT CALLED**   231
By: Claudia V. Francis

CHAPTER 27: **TRIALS TO TRIUMPH: VICTOR OF VIOLENT CRIME**   240
By: Roy Pusey

CHAPTER 28: **THEY KILLED MY PARENTS NOT MY SOUL**   248
By: Dr. Marie Claudine Mukamabano

CHAPTER 29: **DELIVERED BY A SILENT GOD**   255
By: Sashoi M. Grant

CHAPTER 30: **PRESSED FOR THE RELEASE**   263
By: Dr. Keisha Ann Thomas

CHAPTER 31: **HEALING WITH INTENTION**   272
By: Dr. Pearnel Bell

CHAPTER 32: **ENDORSEMENT: I TOO HAVE A STORY**   278
By: Dr. Ernie E. R. Wright Jr.

AFTERWARD   282

CONCLUSION   284

ABOUT THE VISIONARY AUTHOR   286

Introduction

"You can clutch the past so tightly to your chest that it leaves your arms too full to embrace the present." -Jan Gildwell

Intentional Healing: From Scars to Stars Anthology is a compilation of stories of strength, courage, resilience, and triumph through pain to hope and forgiveness. In this volume, thirty-one persons from across the Caribbean, North America, South America, and Europe share how they have navigated grief caused by physical ailments, death and dying, loss of opportunity, broken relationships, loss of identity, loss of one's dignity, discrimination, issues with forgiveness and healing, among other socio-economic and environmental challenges. Unresolved grief resulting from such suffering, inflicted by gruesome social ills, has increasingly posed a threat to human existence and must be treated urgently and deliberately as we treat a pandemic such as COVID-19.

According to Tang and Xiang (2021), "Deaths by COVID-19 have left behind nearly 12 million recent bereaved individuals worldwide and researchers have raised concerns that the circumstances of COVID-19-related deaths will lead to a rise in prevalence of prolonged grief disorder (PGD) cases." Prolonged grief disorder has been a newly added diagnosis in the International Classification of Diseases, eleventh edition (ICD-11). Further to this discovery, a recent study, An Evaluation of Domestic Violence Against Jamaican Women During the Coronavirus Disease (COVID-19) Pandemic by Bourne et al. (2021), stated, "Intimate partner violence has intensified since the COVID-19 pandemic, which means the home has become a battleground for women." This has been corroborated by another study which stated, "Even before COVID-19 existed, domestic violence was already one of the greatest human rights violations." In the previous 12 months, 243 million women and girls (aged 15-49) across the world have been subjected to sexual or physical violence by an intimate partner. As the COVID-19 pandemic continues, this number is likely to grow with multiple impacts on women's wellbeing, their sexual and reproductive health, their mental health, and their ability to participate and lead in the recovery of our societies and economy (Mlambo-Ngcuka, 2020).

While much of the research in this area focused on the relationship between socioeconomic status (SES) and trauma outcomes, there is also sufficient research-based validation, suggesting that early life adversity is a major risk factor for the development of psychological and behavioral problems in adults who experienced childhood maltreatment, classified as Adverse Childhood Experience (ACE). The CDC-Kaiser Permanente ACE is one of the largest and most reliable that was first conducted between 1995 and 1997. For more details, one may contact the CDA-Centers for Disease Control and Prevention at https://www.cdc.gov/violenceprevention/aces/about.html

Why then, you may ask, promote this concept of intentional healing from scars to stars, with a special focus on grieving, healing, and restoration? Grief is inevitable. Despite the kind of losses, our natural reaction is "grief." Be it primary losses associated with significant events such as death and major life changes, secondary losses, as the consequences of primary losses or multiple losses, as several primary losses occurring during the COVID-19 pandemic. Some primary losses are often overlooked because they seem covert at the onset. However, they will subsequently emerge as serious issues and may have a significant impact on one's mental and physical health, which may cause bereavement overload.

Grieving is the process of effectively managing the pain one experiences as a result of any loss. My years of treating the subject of grief, substantiated by the literature, reveal that managing pain may not be grieving. In fact, contrary to popular belief, the tendency to view grieving only as an emotional experience with only symptoms of emotional pain and distress is faulty because grief does have a physical component. The physical side of grief threatens our physical health. Because those physical symptoms can be treated with injections and other forms of medication, one can indeed "effectively manage the pain" without experiencing holistic healing.

Healing, on the other hand, speaks to the process of becoming healthy after experiencing pain. Restoration, which is the act of returning to a former state or condition, is the hallmark of this process and is absolutely necessary for one to experience and live a healthy, fulfilled life, amidst grief. Too often, persons who have suffered a loss are left drifting and tossing in the storm of life and sometimes are engulfed by the whirlwind of life's circumstances, with little or no hope of experiencing any form of healing. Approaching the effective management of grief in an intentional and sequential way, juxtaposed with the healing and restoration processes, is intentional, deliberate, necessary, and is designed to provide an excellent and sustainable means of self-evaluation and self-monitoring as one untangles the web of pain toward true and more complete healing. So, grieve if you must.

With this anthology, co-authors were supported to navigate their way through their pain and write their stories to leave readers empowered and hopeful. These stories are also designed to educate, empower, and instill hope in readers. They also serve as a benchmark to keep you in the game of life. They keep you moving forward and experimenting and readjusting your strategy and your plan of action, continuously looking for ways to heal deliberately and intentionally. You may have felt that you do not have the skills, support, or resources you need. When you read these stories, think of the experiences of the authors, how they navigated their scars, and recognise that you can too. Begin to change your belief system and manifest what is possible despite whatever you have done or what has been done to you up to this point in your life, but don't stop there. You see, most people operate out of their personal historical context, out of the memory of things they have done or experienced, or things they have observed. Use this opportunity to rewrite your narrative. Externalize your problem and enhance self-awareness. Start retelling and stop reliving your story. Here is a guide as you journey along.

THE READERS' GUIDE

Congratulations! The fact that you are reading this page suggests you have the tool that will serve as the major guide.

The stories are organized in two phases. Phase one consists of Chapters 1 to 17 and highlights stories of navigating scars of sickness, death, and dying. Phase two comprises Chapters 18 to 30, highlighting scars from social ills such as intimate partner violence, injuries from violent brutal shootings, sexual molestation, rape, and other matters on which we are too often silenced and kept silent about. Chapter 31 is a brief overview of Narrative Therapy and 32 is an endorsement of this volume and precursor to what's coming in Volume II.

To get the most out of this experience:

- Realize when and how grief speaks to you.

- Know that identifying your scars, treating them with intentionality, and getting to the point of letting go will be critical to your healing.

- Understand that the team of subject experts ensures that the emotional triggers within each story are cushioned; however, something that resonates with your scar may be a trigger.

- Take time to read through the contents page to see the various topics and get an aerial view.

- Schedule time to read.

- Be present with the author and gain an appreciation that you are not alone.

- Reviewing their bio in the About the Visionary Authors section toward the back of the book will aid in your understanding that grief is no respecter of persons. And if they can navigate their scars to be shining as a star, illuminating the path of others, you can too.

- Enjoy the process.

It is our hope that these stories will empower you to see yourself on the side of hope despite your scars. You will be empowered to graduate from the clan of people who become discouraged too soon and learn how to be intentional, consistent, deliberate, and fearlessly resilient. If you have not yet known this, know that you deserve a life of peace. You deserve to be healed from your scars. You deserve a good life. You are never too old and neither are your circumstances too huge or complicated that they can't be resolved with the appropriate help. So, get moving. Set another goal, and dream a new dream of a life worth living. If you set your goals for empowerment, healing, and transformation, go after them with all the determination you can muster. Your passion and purpose fueled by your pain will take you places that will amaze you. Tell yourself no matter how bad it is or how bad it gets, I am going to make it. It is possible for me to heal intentionally, transform my "scars into stars," and live my best life! Be the best star you can be, go heal, and go shine!

CHAPTER 1

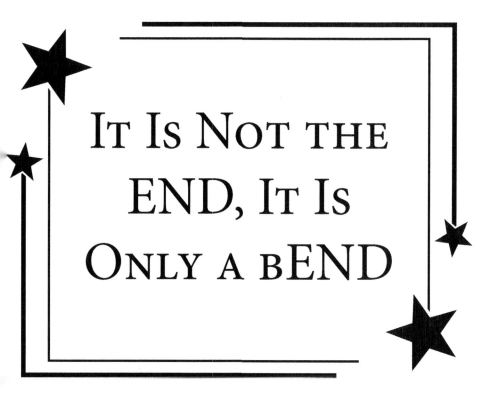

IT IS NOT THE END, IT IS ONLY A bEND

By: **LA-TOYA ARTHUR-TUCKER**

LA-TOYA ARTHUR-TUCKER

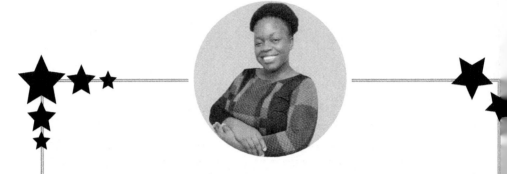

"Consider life's challenge not as the END, but only a bEND."
-La-Toya Authur-Tucker (2022)

La-Toya Arthur-Tucker is a psychologist, educator, author and doctoral candidate specializing in Forensic Psychology with an emphasis in Crisis Response. Mrs. Arthur-Tucker's vision for the world is to significantly contribute towards social change. Additionally, Mrs. Arthur-Tucker is a full-time lecturer at the University of Guyana, Turkeyen Campus within the College of Behavioural Sciences and Research. She is also a part-time lecturer at the University of The Southern Caribbean (Guyana Site) within the Social Sciences Department. As an experienced Psychologist for eight years, Mrs. Arthur-Tucker holds a MSc. Counselling Psychology, Emphasis in Educational Psychology, and a BSc. (Hons) in Psychology, Minor in Social Work from the Northern Caribbean University Mandeville, Jamaica. Mrs. Arthur-Tucker is technically skilled to recognise, diagnose, and treat mental illness through psychotherapeutic, psycho-educational, and psychosocial interventions. She is equipped to motivate individuals to hone their abilities and strengths towards a common goal. An excellent public speaker and presenter, Mrs. Arthur-Tucker, presents at seminars and trainings, both formally and informally. Her humble and intelligent persona allows her to balance family, employment, church responsibilities, and education, serving as a wife, mother, working professional, church leader, and student.

INTENTION

L ife can be seen as burdensome, frustrating and we can sometimes lose hope. As daybreak is immediately after the darkest hour, so is our breakthrough moment. It precedes the most difficult experiences of our life. Reading this chapter, you should realize that twists and turns should strengthen our resilience. You should be motivated to cling to that thread of hope which can be found in Christ Jesus to take you through any situation. Be motivated, irrespective of the outcome of your experience, and gain the strength to be renewed. Ultimately you should realize that your challenge is just the bEND and not the END.

IT IS NOT THE END, IT IS ONLY A bEND

Having graduated with honors, acceptance on a full graduate scholarship was a major achievement. I was motivated for greatness. I was young and ready for the world of opportunities. My first pregnancy was accompanied by discomfort, anxiety, and nervousness for the delivery process. Compared to the discomfort I experienced through the gestational period, the delivery was horrific as the doctors were abrasive, rude, impatient, and disrespectful while the nurses were miserable. At the hospital, it was worse than I anticipated. However, I was encouraged that life would get better when I beheld my firstborn. The experience was awesome. I connected with the most adorable living being with whom I interacted for nine months, finally being able to cuddle, touch, kiss, and feel her physically.

Graduating the following year with my master's degree added much to my joy. I was poised for greatness. All those unpleasant memories are etched in my mind to guide how I respond to the greatness ahead. To add to my success story, I launched my first book, Achieving Success: Never Give Up!, the same year of my graduation and we had moved to a new two-bedroom apartment in an upper working-class neighborhood. Success was flowing. As a songwriter said, "Nothing could stop us, nothing could stop us now." Life was truly great.

We were also positioned to commence the quest for our property. After months of searching and consulting, we were about to seal a deal for our property. This was amazing! My husband and I both held church offices. Amidst all that was happening, strengthening my spiritual relationship was of utmost importance. My social network grew wider and stronger with more positive and supportive persons. Our nuclear family grew from strength to strength. Not before long, Jenae, my firstborn, started clinging to other children at church as she referred to them as her brother or sister. Within a short time, she requested a brother or sister of her own. We considered this request strongly. As we thought about this further, the unpleasant experiences of the first encounter at the hospital served as an obstacle. We approached this with a prayerful attitude and awaited guidance from God. In the interim, we engaged in consultations with doctors and through family planning exercises, we weighed our options. Financial resources were assessed, social support strengthened, and efforts were directed to one goal of family extension. We were motivated and hopeful that my second pregnancy was going to be better. We were truly excited about this decision, despite the uncertainties, we were in for the blessings and expectantly hopeful that all things will be well.

A few things were done differently, the medical practitioner was changed, and efforts to do the procedure privately were considered along with accessing therapeutic interventions. Everything was streamlined and the request was considered. Then it was lights, action, camera, and we were rolling! I started experiencing physiological changes. When the feelings were prolonged to three days, a pregnancy test was done, and voila, I was two weeks pregnant. The feelings were kaleidoscopic: fear, excitement, anger, and annoyance among others. Positive thoughts were utilized to maintain a healthy experience.

Everything that seemed well started taking a turn. Life started presenting some bENDS. Every bEND carried a negative feeling that made things seem like it was the end. Every time, there was a scope for greatness, something made it grow dim. Some bENDs encountered including the living space became uncomfortable, the deal to own our property became problematic, and the seller changed his mind. This heightened my husband's frustration, especially knowing how much was already invested in the agreement. While seeking to manage these stressors, he was transferred to a different extension area on the island with added intrapersonal conflicts on the job. My application for a doctoral programme was denied and to top it off, we moved to a rural community where several things were inaccessible, including the much-needed internet access. Things were not looking good being pregnant.

The second pregnancy brought many scars. The experience started at midnight on October 30, 2016. The signs of labour began, and I moved immediately to the hospital. I was unable to walk the stairs, so I was taken upstairs by elevator in a wheelchair. The medical team was shocked at the size of my tummy being a 5 foot tall, 31-year-old woman in what appeared to be a teenager's body. "I think this woman is having twins," one nurse uttered. As they argued about the size of my tummy, the pain intensified. I was quickly attended to and was placed to rest. No one explained that I was supposed to remain in bed because the medication resulted in me feeling dizzy. After 10 minutes of being in bed, the urge to use the bathroom was felt. Without informing anyone I made my way to the bathroom. Upon my return, I felt the hospital spinning, so I held on to the wall to avoid falling. A janitor recognized something was wrong and reached out to help. "Nurse! Nurse! I need help; this patient almost fell!" As she shouted to the nurse, she was guided to take the patient back to her bed. Another nurse added, "Please ensure Tucker does not get up from the bed; her meds will make her dizzy." After the janitor ensured that I was back in bed, she then asked, "Who is Tucker?" Only to realize, Tucker was already off the bed and had just returned.

The janitor went to the nurse's station and returned with two nurses who seemed worried. They checked my vitals and checked to see that all was well. They told me not to move from the bed again without help. In less than 3 minutes, I called for the nurses again only to find out a bloody liquid was running down my legs. "Active labor. Prepare for Tucker to be taken to the delivery room." I was whisked into the delivery room and things seemed to be getting better, only to realize this was another bEND.

I was fully dilated but there was no passage for Jediel. He was relaxed and was in no hurry to exit the womb. This journey started in the wee hours of the morning and at 12 noon he was still in the same position.

Hearing the nurses give up hope impacted the entire experience. It was then I realized that life is truly a journey; not everyone who joins the transportation will exit at the same destination as you. Some will exit before, and in some instances based on your journey, you may leave before to continue journeying elsewhere. When they chose to exit their journey on the transport called the delivery process, it was at that time I was able to process who was necessary for my journey. With no medical person around, serious contemplations were made. A request was even made for a caesarian section, to which the nurse declined. "You are too lazy." "You are a good-for-nothing mother." "You are heartless." "You and your unborn child will die." Those were some of the comments I heard.

At the ninth hour, a deliberate effort was exerted to focus only on Jesus, this was the moment it was realized that the end was a huge bEND. He reached out and through His never-ending love, through what nurses and doctors saw as impossible, a possibility was revealed at 17:45 and a bouncing 8 pound 7.5 ounce baby boy was delivered through an emergency C-Section, with perfect APGAR scores. This was not the end; it was only another bEND.

For every negative comment I received, I combated it with developing a positive thought. "You are too lazy," was replaced with, " How strong and hardworking I am and will continue to be." "You are good for nothing mother," was replaced with, "I will share this awesome story with my baby boy and others who may have had bad experiences." (Here I am doing this right now. This is why we MUST speak positive things into being). While efforts were started to make formal complaints, these were replaced with efforts to pray for the medical team. "Father forgive them for they know not what they have done," (Luke 23:34, KJV) was most fitting. They all came to apologize separately, directly, and indirectly. They were amazed at both mother and baby being alive. It is never over until God says so. Gratitude was extended to God for His continued mercies and grace; the baby was delivered with some scars but nothing to hinder him from being a star and mommy looked beyond the scars knowing they were preparing her and baby to become stars.

Both delivery processes taught me how to navigate life's difficult pathways. I honestly felt I was going to die in both instances. I had given up hope in the first instance, a doctor was placed to remind me that I am a star. He firmly reassured me that leaders never quit, and I am the driver of the delivery process, they were mere helpers He explained. The first experience taught me the lesson to drive my life with confidence. This enabled me to drive through the second encounter with assertiveness. I was able to appreciate silence for what it is. Being left alone helped me to cling to a hope that only faith could have seen. When navigating a bend for a known road, irrespective of the dismal nature of the road, it is known that it is a bend. However, when doing so on an unknown road, every turn seems like a bEND. I left my second delivery process with confidence strengthened, stronger faith in God, greater respect for my area of studies (Psychology), stronger determination, heights of positivism, and more empathy for persons who feel alone. I also gained insight and strength from the experiences and prayers of my mother, which influenced my second book, From Tests to Testimonies. My aloneness helped me to be stronger; I appreciated every turn with a bEND in my life, knowing only God can determine my END.

Many times, we allow doubts and negative comments to penetrate our positive attitudes. Life can get hard sometimes. When life knocks us down, sometimes we hastily jump up like a reflex. As a teen, I fell in front of many people, and I was embarrassed. I stayed on the ground, planning how I would get up. Amidst my strategizing, help was offered, I accepted, combined these strategies and I recovered well. I liken life to this experience quite often. When we are knocked down, it is alright to strategize how we will rise. While we did not plan to fall, planning to stand and doing so tall will embody our intentions to remain tall. My scarred delivery processes motivated me to be the best mother. I choose to be impactful in all I do. Irrespective of the size of the ripple, each ripple influences movement in the water; similarly I strive to be a ripple everywhere I go. I live with excitement. I share the experiences with them to teach them how to navigate a bEND and to never allow others to determine your end. I philosophize Philippians 4:13 (KJV), "I can do all things through Christ who strengthens me."

While grief and pain are inevitable, remaining with the hurt and pain does not have to be my reality. My third book, Success Amidst Distress: Never Give Up!, demonstrated the essence of being able to fight even after being knocked down. Being the driver of my journey enables me to consistently utilize positive thoughts. I am empowered to choose to heal, be healthy and live my life according to my idea and dream of reality. Despite the hurdles, obstacles, and setbacks, each scar looks like a mess but has a strong message. I have the scar on my tummy that showed me the nurses and doctors were rough, and it reminds me that no road to success is smooth. Every time I see the dents that scarred Jediel's forehead, which was a result of being left unattended, I am reminded of how deep and strong our impact on stardom will be. I have realized we have scars to embody our stars; it was only a bEND and certainly not the END. What about you? What have your scars come to teach you and will you embrace that reality so you can shine like the star you are meant to be?

Steps Towards Intentional Healing

If you encountered an ordeal called delivery, there are several things you can use as you seek to intentionally navigate your situation. The following are the top three that may prove to be most helpful.

Acceptance of the present: Accept your reality and work on it to make it a remarkable memory for eternity. We came into the world alone and at some point, we will be left alone to go out alone. An interesting fact about being alone is that being alone does not imply loneliness.

Analyse and evaluate your reality: Analyse and evaluate where you are and where you would like to be. Be encouraged by this text, "For I know the thoughts that I think toward you, says the LORD, thoughts of peace and not of evil, to give you a future and a hope," Jeremiah 29:11 KJV. This should help to project and strategize for greatness and position you to aim for whatever God has destined for you.

Reflect and adjust: Reflect and make adjustments to keep climbing higher. There is always room for improvement. Consistently avail yourself to find those areas that are roomy. Believe that God's plans for your life are for you to succeed and consistently be on an upward trajectory. Even when things grow dim, it is only to strengthen you in areas you need improvement. God is capable of taking you to and through anything.

Resources

Linktree: www.linktr.ee/arthurtucker

YouTube: www.youtube.com/channel/UCxKjbDmonEJ9p2dOLaUZs3g

CHAPTER 2

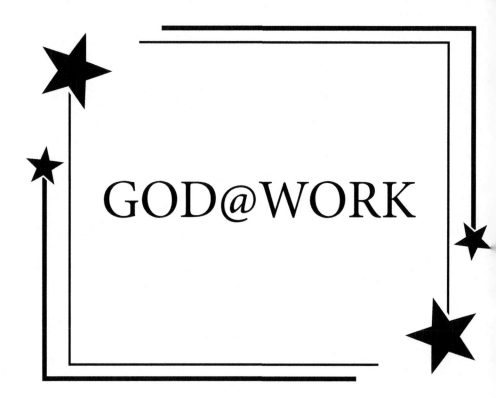

GOD@WORK

By: Jodine Joanna Williams

JODINE JOANNA WILLIAMS

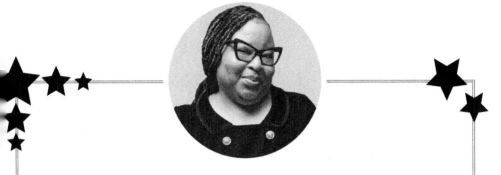

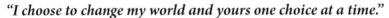

"I choose to change my world and yours one choice at a time."

Jodine Joanna Williams grew up in the rustic rural farming community of Williamsfield on the periphery of the Appleton Estate, in the parish of St. Elizabeth in Jamaica with her parents and three siblings. A graduate of the Bishop Gibson High School in Mandeville, Manchester, she evolved as an active researcher and later grew into a public speaker who has presented at several regional and international conferences. Jodine is a technologically savvy Christian educator with over 27 years of proven expertise in transformational servant leadership and relationship building. She is a fun-loving entrepreneur at heart who enthusiastically reads for experiences and inspiration. She has a passion for life, living, and learning and writes to escape reality and chronicle life-changing experiences for time and eternity. Jodine believes in God; the fundamental foundational value of family; helpfulness is a healthy habit; learning promotes growth, information sharing promotes learning, and that gratitude influences happiness. She also lives her personal purpose which she believes is to reflect God's image daily while empowering others to be the best versions of themselves. Jodine also lives her personal mantra, "Vision coupled with action can change the world," in every component of her life.

INTENTION

Keep your eye on the narrative that God is always at work, even when the sky's scroll seems void of instructions and the sun stands still as a scorching shade. As you read, I want you to note that God gives you quality outcomes through quality people combined with quality processes. Remember, as you journey and craft your story, your outcomes are based on your choices and responses to your people, experiences, and events. You will also learn that you can invest in yourself by equipping yourself with information and surrounding yourself with people who understand you are penning your story on your blank sky.

GOD@WORK

"Here we go again! Yup! That's my name. It's my mom; if it's too quiet or noisy, she calls me, despite having two daughters. I just can't seem to catch a break." Mom's voice was disruptive, plus her lectures and threats to involve dad after work were unnerving. I love my pops. He was the fun but also the feared parent.

"Mommyyyy!" With that blood-curdling scream, I became every adult's focal point. Mom looked annoyed again. But who could blame her? She tried to keep me safe but like Frank Sinatra, I have to do it "my way." Now I was hurting, swelling, and screaming that I didn't see the bees this time. "This girl is going to be the death of me," I heard my mom whisper as she cradled and carried her wounded soldier into the safety of her castle. Cleaned, fed, medicated, and curled up in bed, I cradled my disappointment that today's mission had to be aborted and tomorrow was church.

You see I was a fearless, happy-go-lucky, tree climbing, stone throwing, church girl who lived to prank my overly girlie sister who had a phobia of loving lizards. I played with wild passion and doted on the discoveries carefully nestled in my little world. There was the real world and then there was my world where I ruled like Margaret Thatcher and combed my hair with an unruffled bun to the back like Dr. Mavis Gallimore. In the real world, however, I was the son my father didn't yet have, and the daughter who was poised to be the bane of my mother's existence. I was often loud and rowdy, dirty and untidy with short, tousled hairdos that inspired laughter. But despite it all, I was happy; I was loved, and I had so much fun being me.

My parents nurtured their bundle of curiosity who often ended her days with black and blue blotches, red bruises, and yes like a true warrior princess, a sore foot or two but who's counting? The roller coaster care routine of sleepless nights, church altar, and doctor was as exciting as it was excruciating. Trips to the altar were Davidic experiences where my head was anointed with oil that cascaded over my face into my crying eyes. Doctors' visits were palatable as I liked the handsome doctor who understood and played with me. Mom looked frass one day knowing there would be no school for this melodramatic daughter who woke up covered in blood. Dad's inspection revealed that the oral blisters had ruptured. He was livid because according to him my tongue-sucking habit, which he detested, was causing the bleeding. Blisters and blood were a new feature.

So much for liking the doctor. I had a new doctor who I didn't like. He was all about statistics. Fever, check. Sniffles, check. Blisters, check. Then with glaring disappointment, he told my mom that the sores were because I had placed something heinous in my mouth. Yikes! Even though it was a possibility it was not true, I was sure this day would not end well as I was sick and in trouble. When would this cycle end?

As we headed home, the sun stood still and spewed its vexing venom as we briskly walked the half mile, which felt like 20, from the nearest taxi station home. Along this journey, my skin would often peel, and my body often felt weird. I was no Alice in Wonderland, but I soon decided that there was no place like home.

My condition seemed to worsen; face aches, headaches, and chest aches were now a cause for concern and I had a new doctor who seemed very nice. He was convinced I had an auto-immune disease or two. Lupus and rheumatoid arthritis were on the top of his list, so we needed to do more pricking and prodding. Mom was alarmed. More pumps and pills. Why was my body so disruptive? He removed all my favourite foods from my diet! I had to comply as the stakes were high. I couldn't afford to fail my examinations. "It hurts! I can't breathe! Help me pleaseeeee!" When I revived, I was cradled like a bride in the arms of her lover, but I was scared. I needed my mom!

My medical issues were further complicated by injuries from three motor vehicle accidents. The first accident was my first rodeo with whiplash, and of course, I felt I could easily conquer this thing on my own. By the time I had the big bang experience of the two accidents which happened on the fateful day of April 11, 2005, at 6:30 A.M. and P.M., I had learnt to trust my doctors. The accidents had resulted in lacerations. I had scars but no sores. The almost surreal repeat performance was like crossing the expansive dry land of the Red Sea and Jordan River in one day. To top it off like icing on a cake, I had an asthma attack and by nightfall, the pains were fierce – I was flaring. I was tired! God altruistically grabbed my attention. You see I had settled into a slum where I felt in control dancing at a distance with the Devil and was falling deaf to God's voice. But April 11 was His wake-up confirmation that He wanted my full attention, so He spared me.

My daily delights were my mom's hugs, prayers, and cooking coupled with Dad's encouragement to "strong up yourself" followed by tickles and laughter. I longed to hear Mom call on God as she snuggled me in the warmth of her bosom and massaged my aching body with consecrated olive oil. At home, I had learnt to "strong up myself," push myself beyond my limits, and be discreet with my situation so that became my way of life while I struggled to find direction for the short time I had left on earth. Most days I relished the false hope that I was not sick, masterfully masked my illness, and covered my physical flaws fashionably. But when I flared, with vengeance, I often got to the place where I was tired of the fight within me and of fighting with myself, so in my mind I transitioned into flight mode, flying above the ills and the notion that I was ill. Even people closest to me were shocked when my body publicly betrayed me. I felt slighted and hurt when persons closest to me described my mood swings, breathing irregularities, and pangs of pains that sought to cripple my very soul as psychotic episodes. I wondered if they were right. But my truth was that the more I coughed, the more I cried! My struggle was real!

I was an excellent student when my body gave me the fighting chance to show up and show off. Much to the surprise of many, I graduated with first-class honours from university. I was also endowed with other academic and professional accolades which made my parents proud. But I was also faced with forces that were determined to use my illness against me and it was in the middle of the mayhem that I decided to soar. Despite the successes along the way, I needed to prove to myself that I could excel especially when my body was not cooperating. The pain, anguish, and contention between the cells within my frail frame were screaming for a referee. I had lost time, friends, and opportunities and that's when my central focus on my professional journey began. I elected to invest in managing myself, tapping into my talents, building my credentials, and making my job my ministry. I wasn't sure what that meant but I knew it was time for Jesus to come to work with me. Excellence became my trademark as we became the dynamic duo – Jesus and Jodine on the job but I was still surviving on salvation on the surface.

The inner hostility within my body was exacerbated by injury. God, where are you? You see I had successfully placed Him in boxes. Jesus on the job was scoring an A+. But Jehovah Rapha, the healer, He was my mom's friend and now my praying mother was sick. I cried as I mourned the loss of my prayer partner who was hopeful I would be healed; for now, she laid alive and alert in silence. That's when my 'meet Jehovah' journey began. I met Jehovah El Roi, the God who sees me, through Hagar in the Bible. I became even more grateful for the ordering of the chaotic mishaps of my life under His watchful eyes.

Despite my ugly, I learned not to ask why, as my dad's response was always why not. Instead, I focus on navigating life with my superpower, my auto-immune diseases, creating the best possible experiences for myself and others. I journal, play music, and watch fairy tales as my escape. I find joy in knowing that I have an amazing care team, a fabulous family, and awesome colleagues in whom I take daily pride. I give praises to Jehovah Ezer, my help, who is my Jehovah Shalom, my peace. In my journal, I chronicle with gratitude the myriad of distractions and parcels of hope with which God has gifted me.

Jehovah Immeka, who is always with me, has taught me that the tougher the terrain, the tighter the tendons and the more tremendous the triumph. My journey has been fraught with challenges, but I have learnt that healing is a journey and that the miracle of life is sometimes death, which provides hope and a new beginning.

I have also learnt the value of true conversion and being imputed with His Righteousness. You see, my biggest problem is barricaded by the bricks of my body assaulting and annihilating my good cells, but it's the same body that houses the Holy Spirit, so I leave that seemingly impossible mission to Him. I live with the confidence that Jehovah Elohim, my creator, has me covered.

The most potent language of love is the gift of giving. It is in giving of yourself, your time, and your means that you begin to understand the true nature of a smile from the heart. It's the kind of smile that pushes through pain, conquers fears, surmounts life's challenges, and escapes the lips to brighten a room and warm the heart.

I have grown through my pain. Even though there are days when the flares are vicious, I am no longer a prisoner to my pain and its related circumstances; through this approach, I model to others the value of pushing past their pain. As a team leader and curriculum specialist, I spend a significant portion of my work week leading teams in the collaborative development and validation of course materials, learning resources, and training interventions. Jesus and Jodine are still a winning duo. To ensure I remain true to this commitment, I engage my colleagues and ask for feedback as I endeavour to represent Christ well in my decisions and actions.

God has also gifted me a spirit of willingness, joy, peace, and happiness which radiates through my effervescent smile which releases endorphins that act as painkillers. I know the impact of smiling on my face, disposition, aura, and relationships and utilise it in abundance daily. According to a 2010 study conducted by Professor Andrew Oswald of Warwick Business School in England, employees who smile more often are significantly more productive and creative. So, at work, at home, in social settings, and on the street, I choose to genuinely smile.

Some persons pity me and believe I am a pretender because my scars are invisible, but victory is assured for this warrior princess by Jehovah Tsaba, our Lord and Warrior. Never presume persons are being false.

Some persons like me are consummate at disguising pain from their autoimmune issues and defying the odds. Today, I am surviving a severe case of fibromyalgia, rheumatoid arthritis, and the possibility of mixed connective tissue disease (MCTD). I face each day knowing that I am surrounded by other warriors and I never assume my story is worse than theirs as I am not wearing their shoes.

My mom inculcated in me the love of reading and writing. Find a creative outlet not influenced by social and mainstream media. Live out your story! Capture it privately and when you are ready, take a neon-coloured pen and write it across your sky.

From the very beginning on an open invitation, the God of the Universe took a keen interest in my story to save me. He inserted Himself in every theatrical episode making me a sermon even when I was distracted. This is my sky! This is my story!

Steps Towards Intentional Healing

Life throws many curveballs. If, in life, you have been pitched too many curveballs to mention or bear, you will find the ARC is a point of deflection that will swing them into another direction. Firstly, a supportive and accepting tribe is most valuable. The value of **acceptance** as you navigate the pain space is second to none. Secondly, learn the art of **reflection** as you seek to create better experiences and event outcomes for yourself and others. Finally, embrace **conversion** as a platform of hope that there will be a life without superpowers for those of you who are walking a pathway that parallels mine.

Acceptance: Accept who you are and the fact that you are tied to a care programme, and that flares present limitations which cannot be battled in the mind. When I accepted that reality, it freed me from the shackles of "what ifs." It will also encourage those around you to support your decisions and invest in understanding the fight and flight modes which are crucial for survival and wellbeing.

Reflection: At the end of your days as a part of your personal reflection, note the things eaten, the times you ate and time you took your medication. But more importantly, reflect on the impact of conversations, decisions, and actions on you and those around you. Note the things that require rectifying and quickly apologise or ask forgiveness. There is nothing more exhilarating and liberating than rebuilding bridges or closing chapters.

Conversion: I believe I was created by God so He can fix me. I also believe He is cooperating with science to heal those of us who struggle with ill health. But most importantly, I believe that He can divinely heal us like He did Jarius's daughter. So 'faith' it! Honestly, even though some days I fake it, Jehovah Elnose forgives foolishness and covers it with His righteousness. Strive daily to remain in a covenant relationship with Christ so that, like Abraham, we can end this journey called life as friends of God.

Resources

Instagram: @jaejoanna

Linkedin: @Jodine Williams

FaceBook: @Jodine Joanna Williams

CHAPTER 3

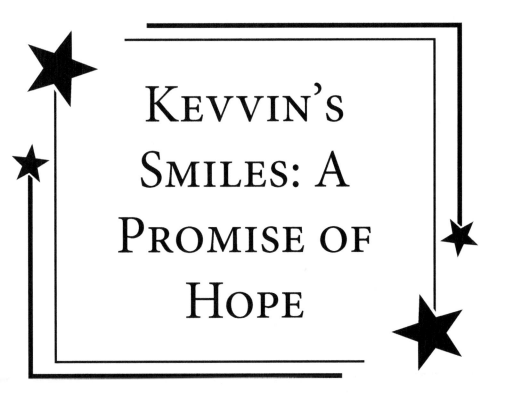

KEVVIN'S SMILES: A PROMISE OF HOPE

BY: **JACKIE THAW**

JACKIE THAW

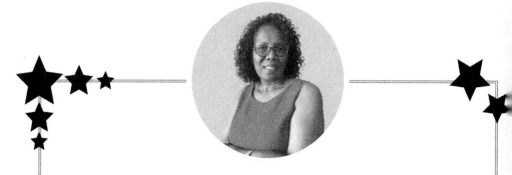

Trust God from the bottom of your heart, don't try to figure out things on your own. Listen to God's voice in everything you do, everywhere you go: He is the one who will keep you on track. - Proverbs 3:5,6 (MSG)

Jacquline Thaw, BSN, RNC-OB, is the wife of an amazing man, Patrick. She is also the proud mother of three adult sons, Christopher, Kevvin and Andrew, and one adorable daughter-in-law, Danni. She is intentional in maintaining the close relationship she has with her extended family.

Jackie has worked as a Labor and Delivery nurse at Hackensack University Medical Center. She is certified in inpatient obstetrics. Her job responsibilities include collaborating with obstetricians, midwives, and other medical personnel to provide evidence-based care in coaching, and educating pregnant women and their families through the childbirth experience. She has received many accolades from patients and their families. She is also the recipient of the National Daisy Award for Extraordinary Nurses. Jackie loves ministry and is an active member of the Lions United Sports Club, based in New York City and travels to Jamaica yearly for mission activities. She and her husband serve as the Relationship Ministry Leaders for their church. She holds a Master's degree in marriage and family therapy and uses the knowledge gained to teach relationship building skills. Jackie also loves gardening. She currently spends most of her time caring for her son, Kevvin, the main character in the story. Jackie loves Jesus and it's her life's goal to follow His lead.

INTENTION

In reading my story, I hope that you will realize that in some situations that you feel like holding on for dear life. You will learn that not until you let go of your own thoughts, feelings, and understanding and hold onto the promises of the Most High God, will you be able to survive and thrive through seemingly unbearable circumstances with the help of the community. You have to let go to hold on. Developing an attitude of gratitude can also aid in lightening the load of life's burden.

KEVVIN'S SMILES: A PROMISE OF HOPE

My marriage to Patrick was great. My children were healthy and well-developed adults of which any parent would be proud. To add to the joy, Kevvin got engaged to and married his high school sweetheart, Danni. In fact, he planned a surprise wedding which went off without a hitch.

I was on cloud nine.

That was one of the happiest times in my and my family's life. We now had the daughter we never had; and for me, I was thinking of holding my future grandbaby in about 2-3 years. The more I thought of that possibility, the grander and more exciting life seemed. I was feeling so elated, emotionally soaring like an eagle.

Kevvin has always been a very gifted child. Musically, he played the piano, saxophone, and guitar. Physically, he played many sports: basketball, soccer, and champion on the track team. He believed in doing his best at everything he put his hands to, and would say, "I have to touch the line." This concept came from basketball practice drills where his team had to repeatedly run from one end of the court to the other, touching the line before returning again. Some of his teammates would take shortcuts by not touching the line before turning around, but not Kevvin.

He has an infectious smile, is very sociable, and has countless friends. As the middle child, he is the bridge between his two siblings. He matured into a very well-rounded, responsible young man and husband. I am super proud to have such a son. Additionally, Kevvin is well-respected among his peers, family, and coworkers. Despite Kevvin battling the autoimmune disease, relapsing polychondritus, which affected the collagen of his eyes, ears, nose, and throat and keeping us busy with doctors' visits, his life was great. His illness was being managed by steroids, which allowed him to perform activities of daily living and gave me hope that he would be okay. Life couldn't have been greater then.

At precisely, 2:30 A.M. Friday morning of September 4, 2020, Danni called, and in the most composed way she could, she reported, "Kevvin said he is having difficulty breathing and I should call the ambulance." In the background, I heard him struggling for air with every breath. My breath stopped as fear gripped me. I felt cold and clammy and all I could say was, "Lord do not let my son die!" I woke Patrick and we rushed to the hospital. Again, "Lord, please save my son's life!" was my constant prayer as we walked into the lobby of the Emergency Room (ER).

When we saw Kevvin, he was comatose, trached, (tracheostomy), and on a ventilator. As a nurse with 40 years of experience, I analyzed the monitors and saw that his vital signs were stable. "Thank You God for saving his life." The ER doctor conveyed that the paramedics reported that upon arrival at the house, Kevvin was having a seizure, for which they administered Ativan. His heart stopped, but they were able to resuscitate him. The doctor further explained that as Kevvin stabilized, they did not know how much function he would have because his brain was deprived of oxygen for too long. An MRI of the brain showed severe brain damage in all areas. My heart sank as the neurologist explained what to expect. Kevvin would not be able to be weaned from the respirator, see, walk, or communicate because all the areas of the brain that control those activities were severely damaged.

He then asked what our plan was. Would Kevvin want to be hooked up to a ventilator with tubes coming from his body? Plan??? What plan? You make a plan for a situation that you anticipate. Who had a plan for this? I answered, "No, Kevvin wouldn't want that, but God is going to heal him." The neurologist looked at me like I was crazy. I left that room asking God for a miracle and a sign.

I felt labor pains all over again. I didn't think I could live through this ordeal. I was angry (at myself more than anything), disappointed, ashamed, and felt like I failed. You see, as a nurse, I felt I should have been able to prevent the medical emergency from happening to my son and that I didn't act quickly enough. I felt ashamed that I failed my son as a mother, not being protective enough, even though he was 25 years old, married, and lived two towns away. I took a five-month hiatus from my job. So, operating like a robot, I would go to the hospital for the full visiting hours, from 11:00 A.M. to 7:00 P.M., go home and get whatever rest I could, just to wake up and do it all over again. I was knocked down. Life felt meaningless.

My constant prayer was, "God, I need to hear from you! I need strength to bear this." There on the door of the hospital was a sign that read:

Soon, when all is well,

you will look back at this period in your life

and be glad you never gave up.

Drawing from the experience of caring for my parents during their final days of chronic health conditions, my family took turns being with us at the hospital every day. They cooked and brought us meals, and the church community organized overnight prayer vigils and prayed constantly.

I joined two support groups: a mental health and a grief and loss group. The grief and loss support group led by Dr. Grace gave me the opportunity to receive the self-care that I needed. It helped me put my situation into perspective. I learned that in loss you learn, so I started asking myself, "What can I learn from this?"

Kevvin later woke up and spoke, though, in an unfamiliar room full of strangers (the medical staff), and it felt like heaven. Patrick and I carefully filled him in on what happened. This progress baffled the doctors. They could not understand such change. Kevvin has had some setbacks since and that also confused the doctors, which led me to believe that God is in control and He still works miracles. He does everything in His time. In the process, I have learned many other life lessons along this journey. Another lesson is how much I depended on my own thoughts and ideas. I expected life to go the way I planned. This situation should not have happened because it was not in my plan. So, when it did, things got out of my control. I finally learned that I am not in control of anything. So, I let go and let God.

One night while experiencing a night of very restless sleep, I woke up dripping with sweat as if I had just taken a shower. My bedclothes were completely wet. I felt emotionally and physically exhausted like I just had a very long fight with a lion. I struggled to the bathroom. The emotional turmoil was as heavy as a ton of lead sitting on my head. All I could do was pray, asking God, "What is this about?"

The internal battle raged on: I heard two voices, one very harsh and degrading,

"Look at what happened to your son. You could have prevented this and you didn't.

Now his life and Daanni's are ruined because of your neglect."

"What kind of mother are you? And to add to that, you call yourself a nurse? You helped a lot of people heal, but you failed your own son."

As more and more guilt weighed me down, I tried desperately to defend myself from the accusation, but I could not speak. But then a soft voice replied, "You did the best you could," to which I responded, "Maybe I could have done more..." The voice continued, speaking on my behalf because I was no match for that evil spirit, "Even if you believe you did something wrong, even if you fell short, My grace is sufficient because my strength is made perfect in your weakness" (2 Corinthians 12:9). I went back to bed and had a very peaceful sleep. I realized that incident was a battle between God and the devil for my life. From that moment on, I knew that God would see me through if I only trusted Him to control my life.

Upon my return to work, a large group of my coworkers had sat for exams and passed their certification in Inpatient Obstetrics. I thought to myself, "I would like to do this, but given what I am experiencing, I may not be able to or have the capacity." I was reminded of Kevvin's tenacity, and that he would have chided me for making excuses. So, I decided to study and retake the test, again. Third time's a charm, right? This time, I was successful, with the help of God and the motivation of Kevvin.

The weight was getting lighter but like a roller coaster, there would be ups and downs, promising and very difficult days. I was at work one morning feeling so emotionally drained that I started having physical symptoms, like hypoglycemia (low blood sugar). I felt like I was going to pass out. I held on to the wash basin and cried out, "Jesus! Jesus! Jesus! Please strengthen me, I can not go to my patient's room like this." Very shortly afterward, I felt some strength in my legs. I walked into the room and said good morning to my patient and her visitors. The patient's husband asked, "Nurse, are you a Christian?" to which I answered, "yes, why do you ask?" He responded, "You came into the room and a spirit came with you. I sense that spirit as the Spirit of God." I praised God and thanked Him for revealing Himself to me. I knew that He was developing me, a person filled with scars, into a star.

In one of my moments of despair, I reflected on why this bright, aspiring, fun-loving, very gifted child had to endure this tragedy. Again, another voice echoed, "Would you have been better off not to have given birth to him?" I answered with a resounding "NO!" and almost immediately started thanking God for all the fun times we had experienced up to the point he became ill. I am also grateful that he is still alive and that there is hope of complete healing.

I am grateful that God blessed me to be the mother of such an amazing young man who has taught me many life lessons, I am happy to say. I am thankful that through this terrible experience, I have been surrounded by the strong support of family, friends, and community. I am also grateful that I was able to come to a place where my hope in God is strengthened. When I look at my son, I do not see a sad case or a reason to have a pity party, but another opportunity for God to show that with Him, nothing is impossible. I remain grateful that I saw a big bright smile on Kevvin's face as I opened my eyes, to this miracle and promise after praying. So, whenever Kevvin smiles my husband and I see

God's miracle-working power that brings hope to our hearts. One such experience is Kevvin telling his dad that he loves us.

Having experienced this situation, I got the sense that I am called to be an advocate to help other parents going through tragic situations with their own children. Two months ago, my good friend's 19 year old daughter drowned in Florida while on spring break. The instant I heard the news, I felt the urge to go to her side and show sensitivity and compassion. We cried together, and there was a safe space for her to grieve. I felt her pain, one mother to another.

Many people have told me that I am an encouragement to them. Others have come seeking support through their difficult circumstances; they say they feel a sense of peace from our conversations. Apparently, I am exuding more patience, humility, compassion, gratitude, and understanding for others.

I have gained a wealth of information that has equipped me with the skills required to support individuals preparing for post-hospital care. Part of a case manager's job is to ensure that everything is arranged so that a patient like Kevvin can seamlessly be discharged from the hospital to a rehabilitation facility, another care center, or home.

Remember the sign on the hospital door:

Soon, when all is well,

you will look back at this period in your life

and be glad you never gave up.

Hold on and don't give in to feelings of despair when life's situation knocks you down. Believe you can get through your scars. Like Jesus was in the fiery furnace with the three Hebrew boys, in the lion's den with Daniel, and in the wilderness leading Israel to the promised land, so will He be with you. Pray for strength to embrace each moment. Believe that God will see you through.

Surround yourself with positive, spiritually uplifting people who will remind you of what God has brought you through and to where He is bringing you. Ask God for the courage to believe when you don't. Call on God in the wee hours of the morning when you are awakened and can't go back to sleep. Read God's promises from the Bible and sing them in songs.

Join a support group where people empower each other. Join a ministry and help people in need.

Realize that you can do all things through Christ who gives you strength. Also, realize that God wants the best for you. He can turn your misery into a ministry. Keep trusting Him and take life one day at a time. One day your darkness will become light as you navigate your scars and become shining stars.

Steps Towards Intentional Healing

As you seek to heal intentionally, know that this too shall P.A.S.S.

Pray and meditate. Learn to pray unrealistic prayers and hold on to God's unchanging hands. Feed your soul on his words.

Appreciate your experience and be grateful. Find something for which to be grateful, especially through the difficulties. Praise God that He is working things out for the best even though you don't see it. Grab hold of the promise that all things work together for good to those who love God.

Surround yourself with positive-thinking people who will encourage you. Join support groups. With the help of God and community, dispel all negative thoughts and replace them with positive, uplifting ones.

Share your experience and instill hope. Your trials are not for you alone. As you successfully navigate them, become a conduit of hope.

Resources

Instagram: @jackie.thaw

Linktree: https://linktr.ee/jackie.thaw

CHAPTER 4

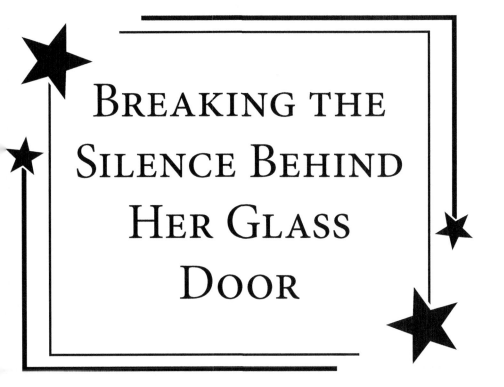

BREAKING THE SILENCE BEHIND HER GLASS DOOR

BY: **STACIA SAMUELS**

STACIA SAMUELS

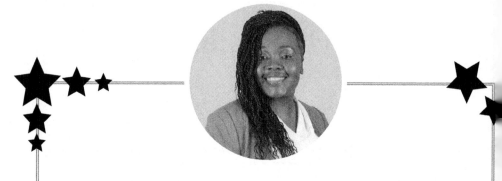

"I don't know what, but I know Who." - Stacia Samuels
"Beloved I wish above all things that thou mayest prosper and be in health even as thy soul prospers." - 3 John 2

Stacia Samuels is a woman on fire for God. She is Jamaican-born, the mother of two, Jaleesa and Jeremiah, and grandmother to Khyrie. Stacia is the founder of Were It Not For Grace Ministries. She also currently hosts an online broadcast called 'Manna For the Soul' with fellow Evangelist Raymond McFarlane. Stacia also holds a diploma in Business Management and is pursuing her BSW from Tyndale University in Toronto, Ontario. As a cancer survivor, Stacia has a personal and powerful testimony of God's healing and His ability to give His believers strength and courage through life's fiery trials. Two scriptures she now lives by are 3 John 2, "Beloved I wish above all things that thou mayest prosper and be in health even as thy soul prospers," and Jeremiah 29:11, "'For I know the plans I have for you,' declares the LORD, 'plans to prosper you and not to harm you, to give you a hope and a future.'" Musically gifted and with a boldness to proclaim God's word through evangelism, Stacia has ministered in various countries across the world including the United States, the Caribbean, Africa, and Canada, and has released 2 albums: Were It Not For Grace and Walking by Faith.

Intention

When you read this chapter, you will find strength, hope, encouragement, and a strong desire to PRESS (Pray, Reconnect, Exhale, Self-Care, and Succeed) forward. You will experience the miracle worker, the divine healer, sustainer, and all-around friend to man, God, as He journeys through this breast cancer experience with Stacia. You will understand who God is to her and the calling that He has placed on her life. As the silence behind her glass door is uncovered, you will be exposed to her vulnerability, faith, and determination to live a positive, inspiring and Christ-centered life.

Breaking the Silence Behind Her Glass Door

We can never run from God's plan for our lives because no matter what, His will must be done. Some of my fondest memories before migrating to Canada in the late 1970s is the time I lived in Jamaica with my grandmother, aunties, uncle, and cousins. It was a time when we lived carefree, slept with our doors unlocked, and windows unbarred. It was a time when everyone in our community helped to raise us children. It was also a time of trust, peace, and happiness. I believe this is what helped to shape me and set the foundation for the person that I've become and the direction that my life has taken. My grandmother not only prayed for me, but she prayed with me and taught me according to the word of God through the leading of the Holy Spirit. Life was sweet then. Some would call them "the good ol' days." Family was family. It was a time when we all looked forward to coming together at church, home, outdoors, with friends, and working together to ensure that we achieved a holistic sense of inclusivity.

If it were not for the love, prayers and care that was poured into me in my formative years, I don't believe that I would be the Stacia that I am today. They trained and taught me in the ways of the Lord. This has anchored me to Jesus Christ. What a wonderful blessing it was to have been surrounded by individuals who genuinely wanted the best for me and made it their duty to ask God's blessings upon my life. I am comforted in knowing that before I was born, God designed me to be His ambassador, His anointed singing evangelist, His mouthpiece. I only needed to walk in my God-given purpose.

There was a great time in my life when God caused me to ride on the high places of life. I shared the gospel music stage with some of the finest singers, dined with high officials, ministered in some of the largest churches and events, and traveled to exotic places worldwide sharing the love of Jesus Christ. My entire life is about unmerited grace and God's favor. It is, was, and will always be about His goodness and mercies running after me even when I walk through the valleys of the shadows of death.

The phone rang and I answered hearing a recorded voice, "This is the Brampton Civic Hospital calling for Stacia Samuels. If this is Stacia Samuels, press 1 to confirm your appointment for your mammogram." I pressed 1 and wrote down the information I had received. There was no fear or hesitation. This was my yearly routine mammogram.

The day of my appointment arrived and I went in expecting to be out within an hour. I was so confident about everything being glitch free that I told my office I would be on time for our 9:15 team meeting. Little did I know that this was the beginning of the journey to the next chapter in my life.

It was a routine examination that took less than an hour to complete. The technician left the room saying that she had to connect with the doctor who was reviewing the images. I got cleaned up, dressed, and was just about ready to leave when the technician returned and asked me to have a seat in the waiting room. In fact, if memory serves me correctly, she asked me if I was in a hurry and would I mind seeing the doctor so that she could explain a few things to me. I paused for a moment, took a deep breath, and asked her if everything was okay. She responded with, "If you have a few minutes, the doctor will be able to explain." I responded with, "No problem, I have time to meet with her." My time in the waiting room seemed endless when in fact, I don't think I waited 20 minutes. You could say that I was very anxious to hear what the doctor had to say to me.

"Ms. Samuels?" "Yes." "May I see your wristband please? I just need to confirm your ID. Okay that's great, please come with me." This time I was taken into a nice little office to meet with the doctor. She was a very nice doctor with a caring disposition. One would say she had great bedside manners. She asked all the appropriate questions and was thorough in her explanations. My family doctor was notified and an appointment was set for the biopsy that started my unforgettable journey through breast cancer.

Have you ever heard the saying "If you live in glass houses don't throw stones"? This is a common, clever proverb that's used to remind people not to live hypocritically or criticize others for a flaw that you yourself possess. The essence of my story titled "Breaking The Silence Behind Her Glass Door" reveals my level of vulnerability. You see, we all have a house with windows and doors; mine has always had the curtains drawn and blinds closed. This part of my journey gives you a view behind the proverbial glass curtains of my home.

Well another famous saying says, "If life gives you lemon make lemonade," and that's how I was forced to live in silence. It was not always easy as a private person having to put your best foot forward all the time, but I purposed in my heart to live in a place of positivity and transparency.

I also applied my P. R. E. S. S. (Pray, Reconnect, Exhale, Self-Care, and Succeed) methodology.

Hearing the doctor confirm that I have the "killer disease" (cancer) growing in my body was a very bitter lemon but nothing that my God couldn't handle. I prayed. My doctor confirmed that with his call on my way home from the hospital. What he said to me made all the difference. "You are not alone." Wow! Who but God would send such assurance to my soul through a medical professional?

The next day I went to see him. He provided a thorough explanation of the report. He looked at me and said, "You are taking this news well." My unfiltered response was, "I know God as my healer." Then I asked some questions and left promising that I would give thought to doing the recommended surgery. He told me not to wait too long because it was in the very early stages and things can change significantly in a short time. All the way home, I entered into communion with the Lord.

A few days later, I turned up hesitantly for my appointment with the surgeon as my preference would be alternative medicine. However, the constant prompting from the surgeon made me pause and ask, "Father, is this You?" I just couldn't understand why they were so interested in doing the surgery. Believing that it was a part of the treatment ordained, I obeyed the voice of God and had my first surgery in December 2020. Was I afraid? No. My relationship with God at that time did not have any room for fear. In January 2021, I went for my check-up and the results from the pathologist and I was told that I had to undergo another surgery because they didn't get everything the first time. This news was a bitter lemon to swallow, especially hearing that they would re-open the incision. I wished there were easier ways to navigate cancer, wounds, and scars. But there wasn't at that time.

I was surrounded by some strong supporters: family and friends. I reconnected. Children of God, music therapy was also helpful in navigating this journey. Some of the songs that helped me through are "The Goodness of God," "Broken Hallelujah," "Amazing Grace, My Chains are Gone," "Keep Me In Your Will," and "It is Well."

I exhaled. Like Job, I decided and purposed in my heart, "Though He slay me, yet will I trust in Him: but I will maintain mine own ways before Him" Job 13:15 KJV. I also applied self-care techniques to be able to live my best life in spite of my scar, finally succeeding in navigating from scar to star.

I remember going through a dark period and driving on Highway 410 in Brampton, Ontario, feeling alone and somewhat abandoned; I cried out to God. I asked where are you God? At that moment He whispered that He was right there with me and I was reminded of His constant presence.

I learned a few years ago that our faith is strengthened when we can praise God through our infirmities. One particular Sabbath, I experienced severe mental attacks in the form of depression when I heard the voice of God reminding me that He did not give me this spirit. I jumped up, went to my music room, and just started worshiping. I sang for more than

3 consecutive hours. The Holy Spirit and I laughed and cried together. Every day following that experience, I purposed to find at least one thing for which to be grateful.

This experience taught me to be more appreciative of God's goodness towards me. Some people write gratitude journals or prayers; I write letters to God and read them back to myself, always giving Him thanks for answering my cries. Do whatever works for you. But NEVER forget to P. R. E. S. S. and give God thanks.

I have had a few character development moments where I've learned to be more compassionate, empathetic, and sympathetic, especially towards people navigating grief and loss as a result of cancer. As a result of this challenge, I have developed patience to love, as demonstrated by God, who loves us so much that He gave His only Son, Jesus Christ, for us, as stated in John 3:16. Keeping our eyes FIXED on Jesus throughout our experiences, we will realize that our characters have changed or improved and we have developed some new strengths and are standing on stronger foundations.

Helen Keller said, "Character cannot be developed in ease and quiet. Only through experience of trial and suffering can the soul be strengthened, ambition inspired, and success achieved." This has certainly been the case with me throughout this journey. I've been pushed beyond my comfort limits and stretched like an elastic band with strong elasticity to achieve things that I have been putting off for a long time, prime example, my writing.

In his book Failing Forward, John C. Maxwell says, "Never say die. Never be satisfied. Be stubborn. Be persistent. Integrity is a must. Anything worth having is worth striving for with all your might."

I will bless the Lord at all times: his praise shall continually be in my mouth. - Psalm 34:1

Now don't get me wrong. I'm not saying that I won't have dark days ahead. No absolutely NOT! But having addressed this darkness with the word of God, I am now empowered to live in front of the curtains and no longer behind.

I now shine my light as a star in retelling and not reliving my story as I share on various social media platforms to impact lives on an international scale. I am also more intentional in serving, sponsoring, and supporting the disenfranchised population.

Through my online broadcast ministry "Manna For The Soul," I am empowering and providing access to information to help prepare souls for this blessed hope of a future without sickness or death. There will no longer be permission to touch God's people. Most importantly, death is but a sleep for those who are anchored in Jesus Christ. "O death, where is thy sting? O grave, where is thy victory?" (1 Corinthians 15:55).

Beloved friends, thanks for joining me on this journey. It is no secret what God can do; what He's done for me He can and will do for you. This experience can be yours with a daily commitment and study of His word and abiding in His presence. Read about it in Psalm 91:1. Our Heavenly Father also desires the very BEST for us. 3 John 2 tells me that the sovereign Lord wants me, Stacia, to live in a place of prosperity and health. Mrs. Ellen G. White says it best.

"We have nothing to fear for the future, except as we shall forget the way the Lord has led us and His teaching in our past history. We are now a strong people if we will put our trust in the Lord; for we are handling the mighty truths of the word of God. We have everything to be thankful for. If we walk in the light as it shines upon us from the living oracles of God, we shall have large responsibilities, corresponding to the great light given us of God" (Christian Experience and Teachings of Ellen G. White, pg. 204).

Steps Towards Intentional Healing

We must believe that God wants what's best for us. He tells us in Jeremiah 29:11 that He knows the thoughts that He thinks toward us, thoughts of peace, and not of evil, to give us an expected end. How can we fail with Him by our side? God wants our complete trust to take us into our future. Stay focused and never forget the ways He has led you in the past. Being thankful to God and P. R. E. S. S. are the keys to intentionally navigating breast cancer with the hope of healing:

Prayer: "The soul that turns to God for its help, its support, its power, by daily, earnest prayer, will have noble aspirations, clear perceptions of truth and duty, lofty purposes of action, and a continual hungering and thirsting after righteousness. By maintaining a connection with God, we shall be enabled to diffuse to others through our association with them, the light, the peace, the serenity, that rule in our hearts" (E.G. White. Prayer, Chapter 9).

Reconnect: Individuals in your network should be your pillars of faith. You need your ride-or-die person who you can call any time day or night and they will intercede on your behalf.

Exhale: This is where we pause and reflect while at the same time releasing all the negative energies from people, places and things in our lives. Say so long, bye bye!

Self-Care Uplifting/Inspirational Gospel Music: Sometimes we have no words to express the deep wounds within our souls. Music reaches deep down, touches the inner core, and lifts us to God. It's also essential to maintain a proper diet and exercise.

Succeed: I can do all things through Jesus Christ, who strengthens me! You are finally at the place of acceptance. You are living, no longer existing. Each day you are committed to being your best self. Congratulations!

Resources

Instagram: @staciasamuels3

Facebook: https://www.facebook.com/stacia.samuels.5

YouTube: https://www.youtube.com/watch?v=y5V1QKnMqEU

CHAPTER 5

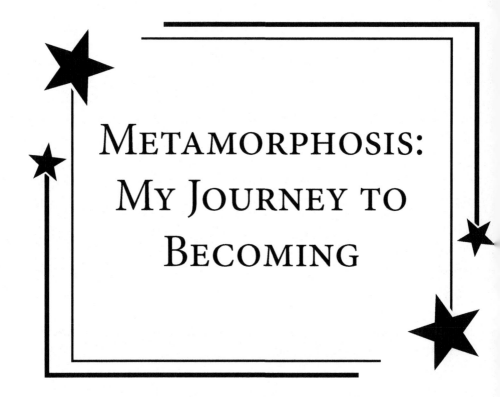

METAMORPHOSIS: MY JOURNEY TO BECOMING

BY: DAWN RICHARDS

Dawn Richards

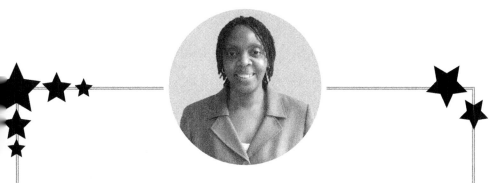

Life – we came into this world for a purpose. Although not equipped with all we need at the onset, it is our experiences, good and bad, that shape us into what we need to be. Embrace them. - Dawn Richards (2022)

Dawn, having attended the University of 'Hard Knocks', now serves as an advocate for attendees. Her success at this institution was accomplished only because of God's grace, which has strengthened her faith in Him more. Her life's challenges began at birth, as a result of illness, but engendered in Dawn a determination to live and a resilience that has sustained her throughout all the challenges encountered in her journey through life. In addition to her life's experiences, and despite the numerous challenges she encountered along the way, she earned a Bachelor's degree in Business Administration From West Indies College, (Now Northern Caribbean University) and a Master's in Counselling from Central Christian University, Sarasota, Florida. Dawn's innate character traits of compassion, mercy, and faithfulness – further honed through the challenges – have led her through the financial sector, early childhood sector, and most recently the trucking industry. In all areas, she has helped to improve the lives and circumstances of others. Dawn's mission in life is to engender hope in those who are in seemingly hopeless situations and help children recognize from an early age who they truly are in Christ so that they will not be hit as hard by the challenges they too will face.

INTENTION

My story was born out of a life of challenges. Were it not for a strong faith in God, I would be walking around as one of unsound mind, but God kept me. As He says repeatedly in His Word, "I will never leave you nor forsake you" (Deuteronomy 31:6,8; Joshua 1:5; Hebrews 13:5 KJV). He never promised ease of passage but His abiding presence. I have come to realise that were it not for His presence, how much worse things could be. By telling my story, I intend and fervently hope that readers will recognize that without God we are nothing and can do nothing; but with Him, overwhelming victory is assured no matter what difficulties we go through in life. Our perspective and focus are key.

METAMORPHOSIS: MY JOURNEY TO BECOMING

Caterpillars hatch from an egg and come in varying colours, shapes, sizes, and textures. They spend the earlier part of their lives stuffing themselves, getting fatter and longer.

I have always hated caterpillars–well most insects for that matter! But I had an older sister who collected them, housed them in jars, and fed them diligently until they transitioned into beautiful butterflies or moths.

Despite my abhorrence of the fluffy little creatures, for some reason, as I thought of composing my story, the word 'metamorphosis' emerged and from there, the life of a caterpillar, hence my title.

Like a caterpillar, the early part of my life into adulthood was spent stuffing myself, not with food, but with experiences that brought much personal pleasure – quality family time as a child, lots of social and church activities, working in fields where I could always improve the lives of others, and networking through the Mandeville Junior Chamber organisation.

There was always something to do, a bit of youthful exuberance, the unrealistic expectation that I was invincible and nothing could ever go wrong, and hopes and dreams were high. Life was great!

Somewhere along the way, reality set in, and it eventually hit me like a bulldozer. In every stage of our development life happens. There were some things I never anticipated, some from which I bounced back quickly but never dealt with the impact and some from which I have yet to fully recover. The amalgamation of these events eroded the foundations of my existence.

People, in general, turn out to be different from the way they portray themselves or how you perceived them to be. The day a teacher, under the guise of providing requested assistance, slipped his hand from my shoulder down into my blouse to cup my breast left me thoroughly disgusted and taken aback. I had never heard of anything like this before.

Then on entering the workforce, I was truly appalled to know that an employer would threaten to give me poor appraisals unless I offered sexual favours. The worst part of this unfolding nightmare is that it was not someone who was free, single, and disengaged. It was also difficult to come to terms with the reality that co-workers and employers would actually collude to prevent you from advancing professionally. As I transitioned and became a business owner, I also suffered at the hands of my staff members as they stole from me, regardless of how well I treated them. I further suffered heartbreaks in the social arena, and I had people telling lies about me simply because they can be told.

It could have been a result of a very sheltered childhood, but I had great difficulty coming to terms with the fact that people were so different. As I encountered each disappointment, my heart filled up with anger, bitterness, fear, mistrust, and the worst ever–unforgiveness. As each hurt impacted my heart, to the point where I could literally feel my heart turn to ice, I decided no more! No one would have the opportunity to hurt me again.

This is the leg on which I transitioned from caterpillar to cocoon.

After the caterpillar stuffs itself, it stops eating one day, hangs upside down from a leaf or twig, and spins itself into a cocoon.

Determined to take care of myself and recover from the effects of life's challenges, I was now spinning like a gig, trying to right the results of the wrongs done to me. I felt totally disoriented and discombobulated. Nothing I attempted seemed to be working, but as I reflected on that period of my life, I realised the failures were because my focus was splintered into many pieces. This was further complicated when I started to attend my current church. I was learning the Word of God. I was excited about serving God, and I attended every church event. It was my view that becoming a "deeper" Christian meant life could only get better. Unfortunately, that was not to be. It was then that things got seemingly worse; I even became angry with God.

The Lord repeatedly convicted me of the condition of my heart, which was burdened with unforgiveness. The message came to me directly, through friends, and various church services.

I took what I believed was the helpful step. I got up each morning quoting Scriptures. This I did for years, but do you realise we can know Scriptures and quote Scriptures but not allow them to transform our lives? Well, that was me.

So, back to that caterpillar.

In that cocoon, the caterpillar is no longer visible, and from what we can see, it is engulfed in darkness.

I was like that caterpillar, shrouded in a place of darkness, a place of confusion, a place of hurt and pain, a place of not knowing how to get back to being on top of the world and in control.

It was on this leg of my journey that the Lord started to speak more forcefully with me about forgiveness, but I refused to take heed. I'm sure He could see how much hurt had been meted out to me, everyone else was wrong. I was not being treated fairly. I had every right to be upset.

God was concerned about me, but He also wanted me to be concerned about myself; He wanted me to see the true condition of my heart and where I would end up if I refused to forgive.

Unable to recognize His love for me, I wore unforgiveness and all the associated negative emotions like a badge of honour, until my immune system was wrecked, and I received a diagnosis of breast cancer.

The shock of this news hit like a ton of bricks. Am I going to die? Where would the money come from for treatment? But God! Friends and family rallied around. The support was undeniable and greatly appreciated. Eventually, though, everyone had to get back to their lives, and then I was left to face the questions, the fears, and the uncertainty on my own.

I decided to do the lifestyle change: dietary changes, regular exercise, making efforts to remain joyful, rest and trust God to complete His work. The lifestyle change worked initially, and I could see the progress; eventually, I was left to do it alone and just couldn't maintain the regimen. In addition, the unforgiveness factor could no longer be ignored.

What else could I do? I followed all the suggestions: I prayed for myself, I prayed for the people who hurt me, I declared God's Word, and I said I forgave, but nothing seemed to be working.

In 2020, someone suggested I say the Model Prayer and insert the names of the people I needed to forgive. I did this for quite a while, and I believe that in addition to everything else I was doing over time, names began falling from my list one by one. The other thing that happened was that eventually, I was convicted that in addition to saying, "Those that trespassed against me," I was to say, "Those whom I perceived had trespassed against me." This was an important transition as I realised that my focus and perception greatly impacted my interpretation of and reaction to my circumstances. Now I needed to refocus and try to get a new perspective on all that had transpired over the years.

When the butterfly emerges from the cocoon, its wings are wet and not fully developed, so it cannot fly. In order to realise its true potential to soar, it expands its wings by pumping fluid from its abdomen through its veins to its wings. Next, it vigorously flutters its wings to dry them and create flight muscles before it can fly. I believe this clearly shows that the entire process of navigating from scars to stars is not an overnight or easy process. Like the butterfly, we need nourishment to be energised with fighting power as we prepare to be airborne. If the process is aborted, we will not become all we are destined to be.

My journey out of the darkness had begun. During the process of becoming, the turmoil is great, the questions are even greater, and the tears were many until eventually I was all cried out. Discerning people around me could see the distress but they also recognized that it would not be in my best interest to interfere, so they gave me hugs and most importantly prayed for and with me. The most amazing part was that on the days when I felt my worst, persons who didn't even know my story would proclaim how good I was looking. "Who but God?!"

In the earlier part of receiving the diagnosis, I was encouraged to start a Gratitude Journal. It was really hard in the beginning. "What was there to be grateful for?" I thought. Nevertheless, I forced myself. Initially, it was only, "Thank You for life," but now without even thinking, I can be in that mode of thanksgiving for an entire day. This keeps my focus on my Father. Truth be told, there is good in everything that we go through if we choose to see it. Moreover, Romans 8:28 (NKJ) assures us that "all things are working together for good for those who love God and are called according to His purpose." This means that even through the bad, good can be expected as the outcome. Of course, there are still days when no matter how hard I try, my focus shifts and the ugly "why's?" resurface. On most of these occasions, someone would call or send a message with just the right words to help me regain my focus. Evidently, the Lord placed me on their heart to connect. So now the down times are more infrequent and for this I am grateful.

This phase of my journey from scars to stars can be likened to the journey of coming out of the cocoon which is also a way of coming out of my comfort zone. Sigh. "Do I really have to Lord?" That's like a rhetorical question, and there are no two ways about it – I must come out of the place of comfort. My arrival at my destination of complete restoration of health and wholeness is non-negotiable.

Even though the transformation process from cocoon to butterfly is painfully slow, our Father stays with us through the process of restoration. It was at that time that my faith, trust, and hope in God, and His healing power grew stronger. I developed characteristics that made me more loving, joyful, and at peace. Those moments of discomfort while navigating my scars taught me patience, kindness, goodness, faithfulness, self-control, and how to 'fly'.

More recently I believe the Lord instructed me to use these points to assess each situation that I had been through and that may arise:

- What personal challenges at the time of the incident caused me to view the interaction as negative?

- What past issues caused me to perceive it as negative?

- What could the other person be going through at the time of the incident that may have caused them to act or speak in the manner they did?

- What may they have gone through in their lives that caused them to act in the way they did?

- Could the weakness I identify in them be a weakness in me that needs to be addressed?

- What was the Lord using in and through the situation to make me a better person?

These questions definitely provided the foundation for a change of focus and perspective. They helped to remove the sting and took me to a place of empathy.

An adult butterfly mates, lays eggs, and reproduces of its kind.

Having survived, and overcome in many areas as a result of this journey, it is only fitting for me to draw near to others, share my life lessons, and pray them through. Daily in conversation, I encounter others hurting, some crying silently, some crying aloud, some too numb to even cry. What else can I do but that which is most needful - remind them consistently that they are not alone, God cares, God can, God will, and His grace is indeed sufficient. On other occasions, someone comes to my mind – more and more I am learning that this is usually an indication that there is a need, and in obedience, I reach out.

When I was asked to co-author this anthology and heard the title, I thought, "But I'm not yet a star. What have I accomplished, and am I yet fully restored?" Then I believe the Lord asked, "What is the purpose of the star?" The light bulb went on: a star brings light in the darkness and provides direction. My prayer is that sharing my story will be that source of light to help others going through seasons of darkness, giving them hope that after each night comes a new dawn. In addition, I pray that my story presents the guardrail that will help someone else avoid- unnecessarily travelling the same road.

Steps Towards Intentional Healing

Ready, **AIM**, Fly!

Are you now ready for the shift, ready to heal intentionally, rise up out of the doldrums, and move full force ahead? Well, let's AIM:

Acknowledge your pain, but don't own it - when you own something, you go the extra mile to care for it to ensure that it remains in mint condition. We definitely don't need to do that with pain. It is holding it dear to our hearts that eventually tears us down. So it happened; remember those questions above and try to work through it.

Intercede - Pray for those involved in the hurtful acts. Matthew 5:44 (NKJ) tells us in part "…pray for those who spitefully use you, and persecute you." This is not at all easy, and for a while, you may literally choke on saying the person's name; however, even years later, you will find it becoming easier to do.

Move - Don't set up residence in that place of darkness. Like the caterpillar transitioning through a cocoon, it is a temporary state to prepare you for that amazing transformation to a beautiful butterfly. Your season of darkness is but for a moment. It is a season of preparation, the launching pad to your divine destiny. You are destined for greatness and you will get there by the grace of God.

Having arrived, soar!

Resources

Instagram: @the_care_centre-jam

Facebook: Dawn Richards

LinkedIn: Dawn Richards

CHAPTER 6

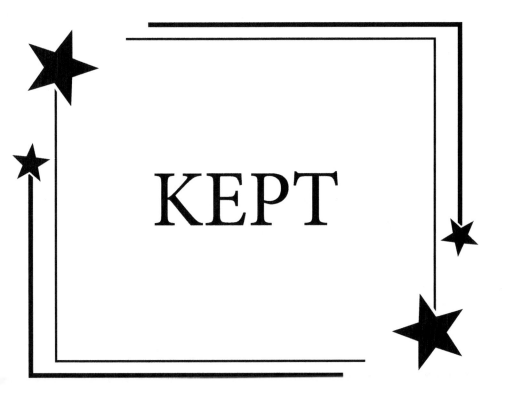

KEPT

BY: DONETTE A. JAMES-SAMUEL

DONETTE A. JAMES-SAMUEL

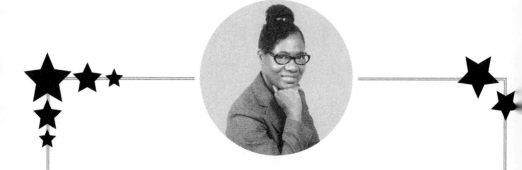

This life is not a dress rehearsal. It is real; my KEEPER is directing.

Donette A. James-Samuel, born in St Elizabeth, Jamaica, resides in England. Life's experiences have taught her much, some of which she shared in contributions to editions of the Devotions for Women by Women produced by the General Conference of Seventh-day Adventist Women's Ministries Department. Donette attained primary and secondary education in St Elizabeth and St James, respectively, and then a BSc in Nursing at Northern Caribbean University, Manchester. She served at the Cornwall Regional Hospital, St James for several years, and attained certification as an Emergency Management Technician from University of the West Indies prior to migration. She has completed a course in Mentorship in Professional Practice at Buckinghamshire New University, UK. She currently serves in the hospital setting caring for Orthopaedic and General Surgery patients. Relaxation involves reading a good book, listening to instrumental music, and traveling globally, including cruises with family. She also enjoys supporting others, particularly her "unofficially adopted" children, spread across Jamaica, Canada, USA, and England. She enjoys choir singing, working with youth, leading pathfinder club, planning charity outreach programmes, and outdoor activities including camping. Her simple lifestyle has not been without challenges, but there are always solutions. One thing is evident: God has been faithful.

INTENTION

It is known that making the journey on this planet without experiencing challenges is not an option. By themselves, challenges are not designed to destroy or discourage, but to provide greater opportunities for advancement and prove our integrity. They dare the ability to remain true and produce a sense of dependency on God. Likewise, not understanding life's events and challenges gives birth to fear. Yet, faith and fear demand the same requirement: belief in things not seen or understood. Faith opens avenues to face realities and rise; let us not be defeated by fear but accomplish great things to God's glory.

KEPT

I was born to anxious parents whose prayers were answered after having five sons. It was interesting and much fun growing up in the hills with awesome parents, siblings, caring family, and neighbors. I was not born to royalty, but felt safe, happy, free, and adventurous. I was always bursting at the seams in anticipation of family times of worshiping, listening to stories on the transistor radio, or simply talking and laughing. I have great memories of being involved in my parents' farming activities; they farmed mainly pineapple. I loved climbing fruit trees, especially mango trees, washing and swimming in the rivers, and playing ball games. A young round fruit, paper wrapped round with a stone at the center for the weight, or just about anything would suffice as a ball. I enjoyed skating in the red mud and dancing in the rain as carefree as the wind. Through those times, God has kept me safe.

School days left their own indelible marks, from running down hills, crossing rivers, to walking five to seven miles to get rides for school when the single bus was non-functional, then riding the train to the closest point and walking another seven miles home. I never had a second thought, but enjoyed every bit.

Years passed, and many more memories were created. Then came true love. My husband loved the Lord, was very passionate about evangelism, and was not shy about that whenever there was an opportunity. With him sharing literature door-to-door and in the streets while I worked with the children ministries and pathfinder, I was always delighted and empowered in the mission of souls for Christ. He was a fun guy, light-hearted and created the space for fun and laughter. When life was great, we certainly had some good laughs at our silliness and even our challenges. I think of special times whether it be the Bible or varying topics of discussion. Times spent in the kitchen when he experimented on cooking various foods were quite interesting because I am very particular about food while he liked trying different types. Going on holiday vacations, whether it was just us or with family and friends, was part of our recreational package. The year before the pandemic, we had an awesome time touring beautiful Jamaica, all fourteen parishes with family and friends. He absolutely loved it. Our relaxing and chilling times were always welcome treats, such as going for walks, listening to music (such as gospel, calypso, and instrumentals), dancing, games, and movie nights.

He was very special, easy-going, and friendly. "A Long and Lasting Love" was rendered at our wedding by my lovely, late friend, Rosemarie, and it was often pleasantly mentioned with smiles or giggles. Lasting love, yes. Long, not quite, but God understands. Earlier years were not without life throwing curve balls my way. I experienced some minor and life-changing events. I had a cycling accident and narrowly avoided motor vehicle collisions, was robbed at knife-point and missed academic opportunities due to numerous constraints.

Then at another flowering, yet crucial aspect of my journey, I made a commitment. Saying I do was meant and hoped for dreaming and building memories together for as long as life permitted, in essence, hoping for a very long time. We made plans, then life knocked me down when the world as we knew it, was hit by a monster: a pandemic that continues to affect lives of every existing human being. By God's grace, we carefully navigated through the first year unscathed. By the second year, we learned to climb on the bumps we encountered. Then towards the end, that monster subtly invaded our home. My gentle giant stood tall and battled. It appeared that we were on the victory path at the finish line, and all seemed well. Within a day, we would have entered the next chapter of our lives when there appeared an unexpected twist in his physiological responses.

In our conversation, he shared feeling better after medical interventions. Urgent investigations ensued. As the medical team stabilized him to get through major clinical investigations, my phone call came. Even before I was informed that he had taken a turn for the worse, the tone of the young female physician's voice conveyed the message. Not much else registered. How I arrived safely, only God knows. My closest family and friends met me at the hospital; praying, waiting, and hoping became a priority for all involved. Denial was my defense.

There was little hope from a human standpoint. As the medical team approached, I felt the intensity of the cold "ice block" feeling in my stomach generating through my body. Their empathy designed to reassure me actually triggered fear, grief, and an out-of-body experience. "This is not happening!" As a nurse, I had been involved in similar situations, but this time being on the receiving end hit like a ton of bricks. The weight of the thoughts and sensations that attacked my body were beyond my comprehension. Nothing made sense, but God controlled my tides. We went home hoping the final call would not come, but it did. My heart shattered into pieces. Why? How? What? Death is so final.

Knocked flat by unforeseen circumstances created the avenue for tough choices. I could either ride the high tides or be swallowed by them. Having experienced loss of loved ones in recent years, I was challenged yet again. Dark days required finding the ray of light, strength, and courage. For some time, the whole picture seemed and felt surreal. But navigating from scars to stars took on a whole new meaning when my dear friend Abigail stayed with me for the first couple of weeks. She was a package sent by God for such a time as that. With a steady head, strong shoulders, caring, empathizing and sympathetic heart, she reminded me that whilst I had to go through the grieving process, the practical aspects had to be done. She plunged in and handled my affairs without reservation. Within a short time, together with my cousin Nikki and sister Beverly, we sorted the bulk of the practicalities. On board were other family and friends in different parts of the world whose expression of love poured into my spirit, and boosted my courage. The support from my church families was second to none. These well founded inputs, made it conceivable to address and execute the necessary plans. I saw and grasped the blessings through the tears.

The summed event occurred nine and a half years to the date of our marriage, only six months to the tenth year. In every waking moment, I was mindful of the turn of events that would change my life forever. During the hours of waiting and praying as the tragedy unfolded, amid my pain, numbness, and confusion, I asked God to make him well knowing all was in God's hands. He made His decision and also made provision. I felt the strain of my nothingness and solitude, but not without the reassurance that God, being my comforter, was keeping me. Even though I don't understand it, I know God does. Before I faced that test, or before my heart began to break, He saw it all as in the past and knew He would have made a way. I may have been taken by surprise, but knowing that nothing astounds God, and He is in control, helps me realize I only have to trust Him. In my feeling of sadness and despair, God has been my joy and my song.

Amid the planning and sorting of final rights, I had compassionate leave from work. Resuming work early raised questions as to how I could have made such a decision at that time. I needed an avenue that could help clear my mind. Hence, being able to change my focus by serving others, was quite the therapeutic outlet I needed. I looked forward to getting in there and forgetting about my worries. I spent time listening to and encouraging others who had much to say about their challenges, whether it be physical, emotional, or any other forms. In other settings, where it was more feasible, sharing thoughts and praying with and for others helped me work through my pain. In those moments, I realized a deeper sense of empathy for others regardless of their circumstances. The heart knows and feels what it feels.

Sometimes my smiles may have appeared awkward. I wondered what others thought when I seemed happy. However, smiling through tears I found strength and determination, although I was disguising my pain a bit. I understood that the testing of my faith would give rise to being patient with myself and others. It was easy to be blinded by grief and focused on my own troubles that I could not see anything else.

However, my focal point was on the importance of spending time with God, lingering in His presence, because He allowed me to see beyond my own trials and heartache to the beautiful plans He has for my life. I believe everything happens for a purpose and God, in His wisdom, permits occurrences. He chose me. He kept me. I will hold fast.

Going through the trauma multiplied my "whys." In my eyes, all seemed well, but then tragedy struck. Why is the first thought, even if not verbalized. Why me? Why this way?

"Why not me?" I responded. Why should it not have happened to me? If not me, who then? I would not have wished any of those clashes of emotions and adrenaline rushes of uncertainty and confusion on anyone. Stopping long enough to change my why's to gratitude, I think of the fact that God could have chosen to take me instead. Nothing is impossible for Him. He could have turned the tide and redirected the course. In my human frailty, remembering to give thanks in all things is sometimes quite a test. This was certainly one of those. However, I am reassured that God knows best. He already knew all that would have happened before I experienced it. I was in His plan all along. When I think of the number of times God saved me from situations of which I have no clue, it is beyond my imagination. With the belief that my situation could have been much worse, I am grateful to God for the lessons and reminders of patience, the uncertainties in life, and the need to depend on Him. I trust I will understand it better, in His time.

What is lemonade without lemons? Challenges are part of our ingredients for growth, strength and stability. Initially, the whole situation appeared bizarre. Nevertheless, upon processing the components, I realized that such events would have occurred at some point. It could have been the reverse, meaning me dying first. When the unexpected occurs in life, the reactions and responses determine the long-term effect. I tried to see the good in the unfavorable settings and sort what action to take to make the best of it.

Yes, it was hard, the emotional pain was real, and it was difficult to grasp. I wrestled with the common or expected thoughts of whether I or anyone could have changed the outcome. But it was clearly out of our hands. I was challenged to maintain self-control and apply growth of responsibility and diligence in relation to all involved. It taught me resilience as I had to reach deep inside for courage and strength when there was only weakness. I chose emotional healing with the understanding that the enemy always fights the hardest when I am closest to my breakthrough. I understand and believe that God sees and soothes my heart, which afforded me the ability to accept my situation.

Going through the grieving process bore no particular pattern. The actual event had occurred, and I had gone through shock, disbelief, and denial. I had to choose to accept my situation to be able to proceed with not only having a life but to live. I have learnt that it will not always be easy to deal with mixed emotions as the memories resurface at any given time under varying conditions. I am often reminded that, "It won't just go away." I understand that, so I have made the choice to live, not just for the present, but in the hope of life beyond this.

I devote my time to working with mainly the ten to fifteen-year-old pathfinders at church. This requires much prayer, patience, sacrifice, respect, space, engagement and understanding. It is as important to them as it is to me, believing that sowing seeds of kindness helps in my spiritual journey and is well worth the effort. Seeing them reciprocate and flourish in that environment, some more visible than others, warms the heart. God be praised! I continue to direct my thoughts in believing the fact that through challenges, faith, and patience, I will see God's promises come to pass in my life.

God has given us the ability to discover the opportunities and power that can sometimes be found hidden in problems. Rise above the obstacles; God does not give us a spirit of fear. Living in hope attracts questions that may or may not warrant specific or straightforward answers, but it is believed that peace and instability are essential for living in this world.

Being tossed by the billows, we sometimes live on the surface, but when we are in partnership with the Creator of life, then we can better understand and accept the pain of reality. It is noteworthy that challenges are part of our spiritual growth experiences. I believe we need challenges. They keep us on our knees and God uses them to sensitize us for works of service. By His grace, we can use those moments to reach out and touch lives in service to God and for His glory.

Steps Towards Intentional Healing

Know that with God, all things are possible. To get through the dark cloud of grief and pain, concentrating on the one true God, can be your greatest asset. Everything He does is perfect. Rest assured, He has His reasons. Persevere through your challenges believing that your God can move any mountain and calm all your storms. You can find much peace, comfort, and reassurance in God's promises. He will never allow your trials to be more than you can bear. He is always standing by to carry your burdens. He says, "Come unto me, and I will give you rest."

Empower and Encourage Others: Redirect your energy to empowering and caring for others rather than focusing on your own trials should give you a sense of worth and reduce the possibility of being succumbed to the human tendency of self-pity. Despite the hurdles, utilize your time by encouraging family and friends knowing that in due course, things will get better and they will learn from your actions to cope.

Pray: When words fail you, entrust your cares to God who knows, cares, and understands your heart. Trust the power of prayer. Spending quality time with Him, even in silence, is the best decision you ever make. He hears the heart and attends to your needs when you struggle to find words.

Time: Spend time on self-care. Listen to music, read, write your thoughts and or feelings, or get professional counseling and therapy. Seek out and embrace the avenues that bring you a sense of upliftment and rejuvenation. Work with that which works for you. Then extend to nurturing others with a level of selflessness. Do unto others as unto God. Through your challenges, allow everyone with whom you come in contact to reap the benefits of the beautiful rose amid the thorny shrubbery.

Resources

Linktree: https://linktr.ee/donettejsamuel

CHAPTER 7

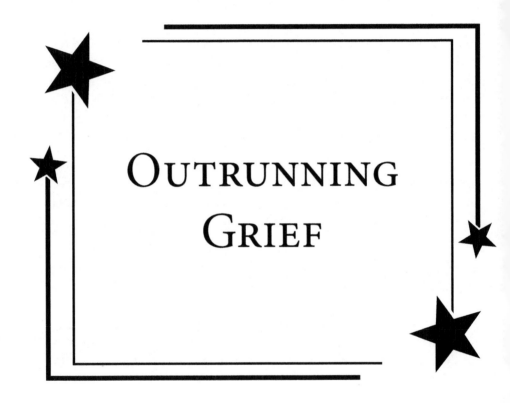

OUTRUNNING GRIEF

By: **CARMEN MAHLUM**

CARMEN MAHLUM

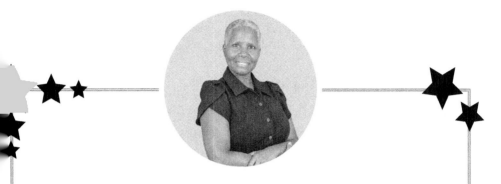

"God is greater than grief! You can't outrun grief!"
- Carmen Mahlum (2022)

In the Fall of 1981, Carmen Reddie Mahlum received her MRS when she married the love of her life, Larry Mahlum. For many years, their work in international development afforded them the opportunity to live in Mali, Côte D'Ivoire, and Madagascar located in West Africa and the Indian Ocean, respectively. From there they transitioned into the world of education which carried them to Haiti and Costa Rica. Upon their return to the United States, Carmen continued her work in education at a midwestern university and Larry became a pastor.

Death has transformed Carmen into a fearless warrior for love! She is in love with life and people again and hopes to inspire others to want to experience love at all levels and to the fullest. As she strives to be present with each person she meets, her focus is not on their weaknesses but on what is good and lovely. She sees herself as the "long arms of love." Love heals!

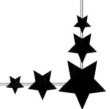

Intention

Even though it may not feel like it, know that grief does not last forever. Journey with me to discover the intricacies of the pain and grief associated with the loss of a spouse. You will realize that you are not alone! Though everyone's journey is different, you must remain open to learning and gaining grief management skills and please give yourself time! The key is to remember that there will be times when you will be unable to utter a single word in prayer, but even a groan will suffice and can be heard and understood by God. My hope is that my story will leave you with hope, a new direction and a deeper understanding of the power of love.

Outrunning Grief

Prior to marriage, one of the most important persons in my life was my father. As I was headed off to university, he made one request of me. "Please, bring home a son-in-law that I can talk to about God." I did just that! My father and mother both agreed, Larry was one in a million! You may ask, what made him so special as a husband and a man? I thought you would never ask!

My life, our marriage, was full of love and adventures! Larry was one of the most fascinating people on the face of the earth. He had a quick mind, spoke multiple languages and was a visionary who lived outside the box. My beloved loved God and people from different cultures. He was fun-loving and wasn't afraid of anything…except for heights. Larry, the consummate intellectual, was gifted with his hands from carpentry to mechanics. He was skilled like MacGyver, the television character who could fix and maneuver his way out of impossible life-threatening situations. If ever one should travel to the most remote locations of the world and experience a vehicle breakdown, Larry was the man you would want to have with you.

Did I mention that he was a banker as well? Larry made regular deposits into my love bank, let me share a couple of examples. One of my earliest memories of Larry's love deposits occurred when we were newlyweds.

One morning as I slowly opened my eyes from deep slumber, I noticed the curtain had been pulled back ever so slightly. Rays of sunlight entered the room and Larry sat staring tenderly at me and said, "Carmen, did you know that you have gold flecks in your skin? Your skin is rich like honey." When he said rich, he dragged it out, as if it was a savory piece of gooey toffee candy…he was almost drooling. Then he held my hand and gently rubbed my arm and said, "You are so soft!" How can anyone not recognize the beauty in the color of your skin? You are beautiful! As a young bride, I not only felt beautiful, but I felt fabulously gorgeous and sexy! Cha-Ching! He made another deposit into my love bank.

One of his most moving acts of kindness was that whenever the baby cried at night, I was forbidden to let my feet hit the ground. He would get up and say, "Ok girlie, get those milk jugs ready." He'd bring the babies for me to nurse. Once fed, he would pick them up, burp them and check to see if they gave him a late-night gift. There were countless times I would wake up to find he wasn't in bed. When I would search for him, Larry would have the baby cradled on his chest as they slept in the rocking chair. Cha-Ching!

We often discussed that if our wealth was measured by our relationships, we were billionaires! Cha-Ching! My love bank was full!

Good Friday 2019 was a fabulous day! That morning I woke up and I made Larry one of his favorite breakfasts. Later, as I prepared his sandwich for lunch, he said to me, "Honey this is the best I have felt in twenty years!" I shouted inwardly, "Yes!" like a bowler who had just knocked down all the bowling pins. "YES! I've got my Larry back!"

In the space of 15 minutes, we went from a fabulous day to life spiraling out of control. In brief, it went something like this. At 10:30 P.M. the cardiologist announced, "He had a heart attack! Scarring indicated that he had had others." At 4:00 A.M. on Saturday, he did what they call projectile vomiting (vomiting that looks like water coming out of a fire hose). They cleaned him up, took him away and brought him back on dialysis. Saturday afternoon he was intubated and "trussed up like a pig." Sunday the 21st, we celebrate his birthday. At 2:50 P.M. on Monday, he was dead!

Initially, I accepted his death. But, on the way home from the hospital, I wanted to return and get him. Reason took over. We didn't go back. That first night without him was lonnnnnnggg! I barely slept. Insomnia was my first late-night's companion for years to come as I kept replaying what he said, "Honey this is the best I have felt in twenty years." How does someone say something like that and then 15 minutes later they are on the way to the hospital? This is the line that caught me off guard and I could not reconcile all that had happened.

Grief hit me like a tsunami. I am not a swimmer. One of my greatest fears is to drown, and it appeared as if I was out in the deep-sea drowning. Anyone who knows me knows that I hate roller coasters! I was ready to get off! This was no Disney or Great Adventures Park ride! I was numb, dumb-struck! My life was shattered by death, loss, grief, pain and sorrow, spiritual desert wonderings along with stormy battering and bruising. I could not pray out loud. My guardian angel had a lot of moaning and groaning to translate. At times, I was spiritually lost wandering the hot, dry dunes of the Sahara Desert. And other times, I was in the deep waters of the Bermuda Triangle like a motherless child. If you were to ask me what kind of music I played back then, I would have said, numb and dumb were the number one tunes on the billboard of my life like rhythm and blues. More like the blues.

Grief robbed me of my identity and sense of safety. They died with Larry.

I was alone! I was angry at Larry for not taking better care of himself for me! I felt ashamed of my selfishness and had a tremendous amount of guilt for feeling that way. How can I as a Christian woman feel this way? Depression set in. Grief sped into my reality like Usain Bolt on the 100-meter dash and I was in a race for my life. I soon realized that I could not outrun Usain, nor could I outrun my grief. No matter how busy I kept avoiding my grief, my loss kept popping up like an angry caged animal seeking a way out. I ran there, I ran here, I did this, I did that, as that was my body's way of dealing with unimaginable grief.

My journey towards healing began one morning after a long hiatus from listening to music. This was something we both loved, and music was a painful reminder of his absence. I instantly remembered the song, "Pass Me Not Oh Gentle Savior." I found it on YouTube, where Fantasia performed it in a scene from a movie where she stood pregnant across the street from a church. She crosses the street, with fear and trepidation, into the sanctuary. With arms raised in anguish and utter helplessness, she sang: "Pass me not oh Gentle Savior," I was in character with her. When she cried, "Mama!" I cried, "Father!"

Her mother began to sing, "Savior, Savior hear, my humble cry." The choir joined in, "While on others thou art calling, do not pass me by." As the congregation laid hands on her and her mother, It was as though "I was her!" I finished singing the verses, prayed, and asked God to heal my wounded broken spirit and save me by His grace. This was the first time after Larry's death I really listened to music. Like Fantasia, I too was pregnant! No, not with a baby, but with grief, loss, pain, sorrow, and fear. She needed her mama, and I, my Heavenly Father.

That day, I stopped running! As Fantasia chose to take the brave steps across the street to healing, I realized her walk was my symbolic walk. I chose healing instead of grieving. The words from Jeremiah 29:11 came to me: "'For I know the plans I have for you,' declares the Lord, 'plans to prosper you and not to harm you, plans to give you hope and a future.'" Well Lord, no more running, I yielded.

A few days later a friend introduced me to Redemption Praise Temple, an online church in New York, where I found community again. I belonged! I found love and God again!

With that, I continued to pray and asked God to "restore my soul" (Psalm 23:3) and "renew a right spirit within me" (Psalm 51:10). I prayed that Jesus would become the center of my joy again. I told God if he's still in the sparrow-watching business, then this little birdie is here. I claimed the gifts of the verse that says, "God has not given us a spirit of fear but of power." I boldly claimed the power, love, and sound mind promised in 2 Timothy 1:7. I tried to memorize Bible verses but discovered my memory had been short-circuited by grief. So, I wrote the verses on 3x5 cards and took them wherever I went. I read them when the spirit of fear rose like a marauding animal ready to devour me.

I also identified the synonyms and antonyms of the word fear. As I read them, I noticed that I had a sad and depressed reaction to the synonyms of fear. And with the antonyms such as courage, and fearlessness, my spirit soared and I experienced peace. Regular exercise was also part of the strategy to deal with the associated stresses. I walked anywhere from 45 minutes to 1.5 hours each day. Walking with my dear friend and prayer helped me to reconnect with nature and appreciate God's handiwork. I was grateful to have a God who loved me! I was happy to be alive again. This time my running wasn't from grief but running to God.

I was no longer interested in asking why, Larry. Instead, I celebrated the fact that I was blessed to have had him as my husband, my best friend, my lover, and my protector. I was grateful he was no longer in pain and I was able to keep my promise that he would not die trussed up like a pig but die with dignity. He lived a life full of love and service for others. My love bank was full, that love fueled me to want to do and be more. Recently, it was as though I heard him say to me, Carmen are you living an abundant life? That propelled me to keep my promise of writing our story. Because of him, I have wonderful children, grandchildren, and great-in-laws who love me. My life is richer for the adventures, conversations, and love we shared.

When I couldn't outrun grief, I found inspiration from nature as I stood on a balcony overlooking the Caribbean Sea. I spotted a lone tree. I was mesmerized by it. It looked battered and bruised, much like me. I captured my experience and transformation in my journal and wrote "The Majestic Tree." This is the best expression of who I have become as a result of my grief journey.

The Majestic Tree

The Tree stood tall and majestic on the outcropping of a hill.

Taller than all the other trees.

How beautiful!

It had withstood many storms.

Alone it stood as a sentinel of the hills.

Resilient!

Magnificent!

Why did that tree captivate me?

Why was it taller than all the others?

I scanned the hill wondering,

Where were all the other trees of its kind?

I wondered how it got there.

How did it come to be planted here?

It reminded me of Africa.

There were lots of questions about the tree, but

At last, I realized the tree took root where it was planted.

Its wind-whipped branches had most of its leaves shorn off.

It looked like it had fought many stormy battles.

Nevertheless, it stood.

That tree reminded me that it takes courage to stay alive.

I could hear it say, "Bring it! I am still standing.

I heard the message from the tree.

Peace washed over me. And then I

heard Louis Armstrong singing in my head,

"And I said to myself, 'What a wonderful world!"

It is indeed a wonderful world!

At that moment, I wanted to be a part of life again.

I caught my breath that day.

Breathe, breathe!

Breathe in what is lovely!

Breathe out what is ugly!

Grief will blow in again with another storm.

But the tree inspired me to stand where I am planted.

Bend if I must but not break.

Like the tree on the knoll, I am still standing.

Standing because life is grand!

-Carmen Mahlum (2022)

Intentional Healing: From Scars to Stars

Though I am still under construction, I want to help others find hope, love, encouragement, and empowerment through my future books as well. I want to see people healed because they learned how to treat their grief.

My encouragement to you as you read is that you give yourself time to grieve and don't compare yourself to anyone. Your journey is your own. Schedule time for grieving, which is a life-changing concept and tool that I took away from the book entitled Grieve If You Must by Dr. Grace Kelly. Her book is chock full of useful knowledge and techniques that I wish I had learned earlier. I recommend you purchase a copy, use it, and trust the process.

Steps Towards Intentional Healing

Stop and be still! Breathe! Don't run from grief! Don't delay treating grief and stop calling it "my grief." Embrace these steps to move intentionally towards healing.

Remember you cannot outrun grief. But you can manage and eventually master grief. Acknowledge and treat your grief. Pray for unwavering intrepid faith. Self-care is an essential tool for recovery. Be gentle with yourself. Speak kindly, comfort yourself as you would other people. It's alright to focus on you now; it's not selfish! Be sure to laugh because it is good medicine.

Learn to think about things that bring you joy. Consider learning something new like painting, writing, and doing more walking. Whatever "it" may be, stretch yourself intellectually, physically, emotionally, and spiritually.

Journaling or writing therapy is helpful. Writing allows you to look back and see how far you have come and offer encouragement as well as a recorded history of your journey. Memory loss is real!

As someone who was swept away by grief and redeemed by love, I encourage you to choose love and live. Reclaim your life! This is what God and your loved one would want for you. Pray! Stand! Remember God is greater than grief! As another dear friend says all the time, "Lean in and trust the process!" I did and it was worth it! You will find meaning and life worth living again!

Resources

Twitter: Mahlum@CarmenMahlum

Instagram: carmen_mahlum923

Facebook: Carmen Reddie Mahlum

CHAPTER 8

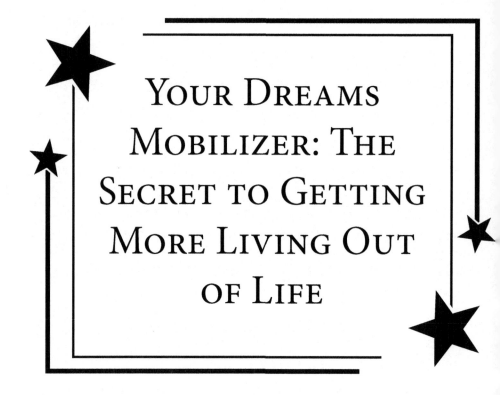

YOUR DREAMS MOBILIZER: THE SECRET TO GETTING MORE LIVING OUT OF LIFE

BY: MELVA SLYTHE-FARQUHARSON

MELVA SLYTHE-FARQUHARSON

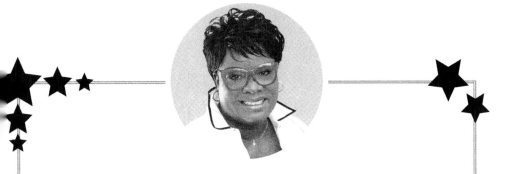

A Dream Mobilizer actively goes after dreams despite and inspite of the obstacles they may face. - Melva Slythe-Farquharson, 2022

Melva Slythe-Farquharson, CEO and Founder of Become With Melva Coaching and The R.I.C.H Mindset Leaders Academy - a scientific program that takes the guesswork out of goal achievement, is a Multi-Million Dollar Independent Sales Director in a Direct Sales Company earning prestigious trips around the world. She is a two-time recipient of the Go-Give Award, the highest award at Mary Kay Inc. Recipients of this award qualify because of unselfish contributions to the advancement of others. Additionally, she has been awarded the Coretta Scott King Memorial Award from the Philadelphia Council of Clergy for her contributions to the empowerment of business owners in the Philadelphia Area. A certified Proctor Gallagher Institute Consultant, Melva facilitates Thinking Into Results (TIR), a program on the science and mechanics of goal achievement. Melva now lives the life she dreamt of, with her two children, her mom and with her friend, soulmate and 'omega' man-Devon, while serving thousands as an internationally acclaimed Dream Mobilizer.

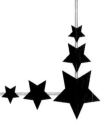

INTENTION

It is my intention to bring awareness to the power of our marvelous minds. When you are conscious of the way your mind works, you will be surprised at how equipped you are to   enjoy harmonious relationships and go after your dreams. It is significant to note that you can get more living out of life only through pursuing your dreams.

YOUR DREAMS MOBILIZER: THE SECRET TO GETTING MORE LIVING OUT OF LIFE

Most people hold a mental picture of the good life! Such images usually form the perceived idea of right and wrong and what constitutes happiness. I am no different. Even as a little girl, I had a dream of the good life which included being rich, successful, owning a mansion and no financial burdens.

My childhood in Jamaica included trekking barefooted by choice and selling apples at school while my classmates played. These are some of my fondest memories but at the time I did not realize I was poor. When I think of my uncle and the fact that he had the criteria of what I thought made up the good life, I recognized my poor state. He had far more space than he needed! I wanted to live like that someday. Uncle was a respected and smart worker who believed in giving. He became my role model and his attitude to life was the catalyst for who I am today. He practiced the concept "Paying It Forward", a concept that I have adopted and adapted in my own life.

I remembered clearly that it was mid-summer in New York and, as hot as it was outside, the heat could not compare to the blazing fire of excitement within me. Our team closed the year with a million-dollar sales record. It was the first that a Jamaican native led a team to such success. This could not have been achieved without my dependable Executive Assistant, Lois, and the other team members. Lois was a strategist, a motivator, and the most authentic friend I could have. We would sing our hearts out with songs that celebrated our achievements.

Our consistent business success, as a top-producing organization in direct sales, afforded us the privilege to purchase our second home in the hills of Pennsylvania. Finally, I was able to meet one of the criteria for living the good life: owning a mansion. Located beside a golf course, this mansion was architecturally elegant with cathedral ceilings, a dual staircase, a study off the master bedroom, a prayer room, a three-car garage, an office, and en suite bathrooms. We shared our acquired dream and success by hosting business meetings within the walls of our home, fully giving others the experience and inspiration of acquired dreams so that they too will pursue their dreams until they become acquired dreams. Once, at a family reunion, my grandma Lady Dunstan tried to convince me to use the garage as a retail space. To her, it seemed as if we had more room than we needed and in her best Jamaican voice, she declared, "Why yuh doan turn dis into a shop!" (Why not turn this space into a store?)

Excellence in sales was incentivised with a trip each year. Another criterion for living the good life was met: The ability to travel the world. My most memorable of which was Stockholm, Sweden where we stayed at the Grand Hotel. The stately decor of the hotel created a regal ambiance. It was perched alongside the river overlooking the castle. It was during dinner at City Hall, the place where the Nobel Peace Prize was held, I became conscious of the turn my life had taken. My lips paused in gratitude to God. My heart surrendered in profound humility.

"Whatever your mind can conceive and believe you can achieve." Napoleon Hill

I learned how to manifest a successful business, a dream home, and amazing relationships by mobilizing my dreams. Jesse Jackson says it best "You cannot teach what you do not know, you cannot lead where you do not go." I live the life and I am qualified to teach others how to live the life.

Walking with my mother was always an adventure. These walks held conversations between best friends. I never allow myself to think of not having her around. Spring 2006 hit me with that very possibility. It was the sound of groaning that awoke me to the fact that something was drastically wrong. Ironically, it was just before dawn. Even the weather was echoing the tragedy I was facing. My mother resembled a spool of thread having no desire to be unraveled. She sheepishly shared her distress and no time was wasted in calling the paramedics. As the hour got darker so was the news delivered by the doctors. It was emergency surgery and hospitalization that lasted for months. The longest two and half months I have ever faced and have no desire to face such again. The circle of life is one of life and death. At the forefront of my thoughts was the question, "Am I about to lose my mother as I get ready for the birth of my second child?" Life has a way of parallelling good and bad, joy and sorrow. I lost my grandfather two days after I sat my entrance exam for high school and I lost my favorite uncle while I was pregnant with my first son. "No, not again! I can't accept such a situation."

Mother kept having frequent hospital stays. My maternal grandmother died in Jamaica that fall, severing the glue that held our relatives together, as well as my hope for family cohesion. I had the sacred honor of painting her tomb. The intensity of each stroke of the brush was a deep desperate cry for harmony. Five months later and I was forced to read the scripture "O death, where is thy sting? O grave where is thy victory?" 1 Corinthians 15:55 KJV It was the funeral service of my father, a father I thought I needed more time to know.

After the tragedies and near tragedies, I returned home to Pennsylvania and a business suffering from neglect and much-needed attention. My first thought was how much more loss could I take? Was my business a part of the tragedy or near tragedy? We started having more months than money, my marriage gradually imploded, both homes had to be sold and relocation was imminent. Feelings of loss, anger, confusion and anxiety fought for dominance in my mind. Sleepless nights led to tiresome mornings. The act of pulling the sheets over my head was my great escape from reality. I was in depression mode. Why is it that in the midst of joy, sorrow rears its ugly head? My unsettling negative interpretation of, "to whom much is given much is required" was about to become my constant companion.

After every night there is a morning. There is a cloud with a silver lining. The rainbow comes after the rain. What if life is happening for you and not to you?

This provocative question rolled over and over in my mind like the tires of my SUV rolled down the highways. The destination was twelve hours of driving to Florida. The trip was amazing and cathartic. The scenery was beautiful and calming. If I were a device, that trip would be a reset.

Mom, my best friend, sat in the passenger seat looking like an escaped hostage. She was unfamiliar with the new me: scared pessimist, having lost my confidence and zeal. She, on the other hand, never lost faith and stayed constant in prayer. I was crying inside and when I could not hold the tears anymore, hope came in the scripture "Behold, I will do a new thing; now it shall spring forth; shall you not know it? I will even make a way in the wilderness, and rivers in the desert. I will do it" Isaiah 43:19-20 KJV This shifted my awareness, inspiring me into positive self-talk. I regained my optimism.

A day later we were in Florida reinventing ME. I did a total self-analysis, assessing whether or not I acted against the best interests of my children, my physical and mental well-being, and my relationship with those I encounter. That small, still voice directed me to harvest the good. I had to acknowledge the lessons that contributed to my happiness and recognize that the past is part of the lesson but should remain in the past. The key to being a successful dream mobilizer is to stay focused on renewal of self and relationships.

Having a passion for empowering others to rise from their ashes, believe in themselves and mobilize their dreams became personal and purposeful. First I had to rework my own self-image according to Maxwell Maltz teachings, "You cannot outperform your self-image." A new approach had to be taken for service: being deliberate and striving for personal development. It was not easy to overcome the brokenness I faced or shed the pain of losses. I had to forgive everyone, especially myself. It was only through the forgiveness of self that I was able to embrace the love from another and open my heart to a new loving marital relationship, where I found a friend, a soulmate, and an 'omega' man.

Experimenting, guessing, or going it alone is not an option for a better experience. I choose elite coaching, study, implementation, and collaborating with like-minded individuals for personal growth and development. Finding Melva who was qualified to be a Dream Mobilizer was not an easy task. The Proctor Gallagher Institute TIR process was instrumental in guiding the way to self-mastery and transformation. Self Mastery is an ongoing process. A close friend once shared that the only directive to pay comes from the statement PAY ATTENTION. Paying attention to your fears and your results are great indicators to where you can grow. Being a part of the process of writing for this anthology has also opened my eyes to the many scars I bore and equipped me with additional tools to heal intentionally. I victoriously clutched my scars, added the adhesives of unconditional love, and let in the light that continues to guide me to my north star.

A shift in mindset is the key to mobilizing your dreams. There were times I experienced pulling the sheets over my head, not wanting to face a new day. There were times when I had sleepless nights which left me more tired than rested. Armed with a Melva Machine paradigm shift, a new way of thinking became my most valuable treasure. To wake each morning to a breath of fresh air is now a gift. It is a nod to continue the work of helping others accomplish their dreams. "Whatsoever things are true, whatsoever things are honest, whatsoever things are just, whatsoever things are pure, whatsoever things are lovely, whatsoever things are of good report; if there be any virtue and if there be any praise, think on these things." Philippians 4:8 KJV

Cycling through limitations, abundance, losses and pain back into prosperity thinking has strengthened my desire to help others mobilize their dreams. The highlight of life is listening to people paint the picture of the life they really want to live. It is seeing the ear-to-ear smiles on their faces and the joy their families experience when those pictures become real. Priceless!

Sometimes we meet people who give so much more than they are capable of receiving. We are apt to judge them. We take their sweetness for weakness. What we may not realize is that their bout with poverty taught them 'giving'. As it is written, it is more blessed to give than to receive. Their desire for prosperity is intertwined with their passion for helping others.

From my childhood, I wanted to experience a life of prosperity with an addendum to ensure the actions I take would benefit others. It was a promise to myself. That is what my third-grade teacher, Mrs. Haye, did for me when she admonished our class to save. Since I did not have money to save, I came up with the idea to sell the apples that I often ate for lunch to make money. It was the start of my entrepreneurial pursuit, creativity and courage.

It is said that experience teaches wisdom. I want to politely add that our experience also builds character. I learned to practice unconditional love for all when I lost my dad. I learned forgiveness, kindness and selflessness after my divorce and I gained the courage to move forward.

I am grateful for the challenges that I have met which molded and transformed me into becoming a Dream Mobilizer. As a result of this empowerment, I have created opportunities for hundreds to experience the mindset shift from poverty to prosperity. Helping them navigate from a life of struggle to a life of accomplishment has been the greatest feeling in this cycle of life. To see someone getting more living out of life is a reward in itself. My commitment moving forward is to continue helping people mobilize their wildest dreams and get more living out of life, which is being realized through my Independent Mary Kay business, Become With Melva Coaching Program and The R.I.C.H Mindset Leaders Academy.

As we grow in awareness, we find that we are only a thought away from creating new feelings which leads to taking actions that can culminate in satisfying results. Nothing is either good or bad, only thinking makes it so. You should learn the lesson and harvest the good. Wayne Dyer says it best, "If you change the way you look at things, the things you look at changes." I received a card years ago and it was inscribed with these words:

"I have a premonition that soars on silver wings.

It is a dream of your accomplishments of many wondrous things.

I do not know beneath which sky or where you will challenge faith.

I only know it will be high!

I only know it will be great."

-Anonymous

INTENTIONAL HEALING: FROM SCARS TO STARS

Steps Towards Intentional Healing

As you seek to intentionally heal, navigate from scars to stars and mobilize your dreams, here are six steps:

Dream: Dreams are meant to grow you. What do you want to be, do, have or give? Without a vision, the people perish" (Proverbs 29:18 KJV). Accept the idea that it is worth going after your dream.

Results: Write a script of your life the way you want it to be. Invite your imagination to partner with you. Use the theater of your mind and act your role as the star of your life movie. Immersively visualize this amazing outcome for your life until it is so.

Empowering Questions: Ask empowering questions that will guide you to finding the way forward, questions that will engage you in exploring whether your thinking is serving your greatest good.

Action: Infuse daily actions like consistent study, exercise, repetitive writing of your goal, prayer and meditation, affirmations, gratitude, sending love to your pain and a positive revision of your day before bed.

Mentorship & Mastermind: I love Bob Proctor's definition of a mentor as someone who sees more talent and ability within you than you see in yourself and helps bring it out of you. Invest in a coach and join a mastermind group.

Self-Image: You can easily evaluate the image you are entertaining in any area of your life based on your results. Continuously improve your self-image. Dress and act like the person you want to become. You cannot outperform the image you hold of yourself.

Mobilize your dreams! It's the catalyst for getting "more living" out of life. Life is too short to wait to be great!

Resources

Website: www.becomewithmelva.com

Facebook: https://facebook.com/groups/dreamsmobilizer

CHAPTER 9

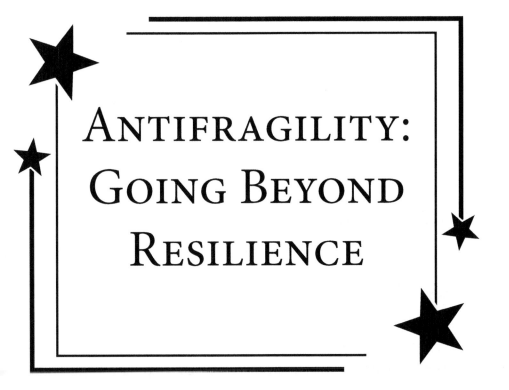

ANTIFRAGILITY: GOING BEYOND RESILIENCE

By: **TISHAUNA MULLINGS**

TISHAUNA MULLINGS

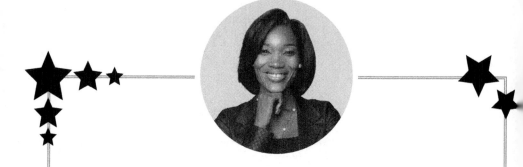

You can build your mental muscles to become antifragile with the right kind of support. - Tishauna Mullings (2022)

Tishauna Mullings is a social entrepreneur with a diverse background having worked in the financial services sector, community development, and the agricultural sector. Though her background is multifaceted, there has always been one central theme in her work: community wealth building through rural regeneration. Her work has seen her serving in national roles such as Ambassador for the National Financial Inclusion Strategy for the Bank of Jamaica and National Farm Queen 2014, becoming an example of success in her locality. In May 2019, she received an award for being one of the 30 most influential young leaders under 30 of Caribbean American Heritage from the Institute of Caribbean Studies. These experiences now inform the corporate training and educational services offered through her social enterprise: NexxStepp Lifelong Educational Services. This social enterprise, located in St. Thomas, Jamaica, serves hundreds of youth and adults with life-transforming work experience opportunities and has received awards from USAID and other local and international bodies for work in rural regeneration. Tishauna completed a Bachelor's degree in Psychology at the Northern Caribbean University and a Master's degree in Development Administration and Planning at the University College of London with a mission to position the social enterprise sector as an avenue to regenerate rural communities to facilitate sustainable development in Jamaica and in the diaspora. Having completed post-graduate studies in Education and Training, she executes coaching and training programs insightfully helping scores of clients to access their greatest potential, grow their organisations, and transform their communities.

Intention

As human beings, we respond differently to various occurrences in our lives. If five persons have the exact experience, it is likely that their responses will be different. Some will grow from it while others experience a crippling kind of gloom. It is possible to not only stay resilient throughout our challenges, but we can actually become better and grow stronger as we unlock the gifts that the healing from grief brings. Journey with me as you will see how experiencing the death of a loved one can open a door that can lead you to rock bottom; with support from colleagues and friends, you can find an empowering perspective and be able to find "gems" in this moment of grief.

Antifragility: Going Beyond Resilience

Ever since I was aware of who I was, I had a sense that I was special and felt that there were unique gifts that I carried that could change the world. Even before I could understand what the gifts were and how they could change the world, I was aware that the gifts were somewhere deep on the inside. I was ushered into a very interesting life as the first child to my mother and the eleventh of twelve children for my dad. I have often likened myself to Joseph in the Bible as he was the first child for his mother Rachel and the eleventh son for his father Jacob. He was seen as having the blessing of fruitfulness on his life and wore a coat of many colours to symbolise his birthright. I was exposed to the church very early. I found great joy in Bible stories and started drawing meanings for my own life from a very young age. So, I grew up believing I was blessed to be as fruitful as Joseph and was very fascinated by the coat of many colours. So as I grew older and wiser, I developed the conviction over time that all things would work out for my good like it did for Joseph.

As the first child for my mom, she had the joy of buying clothes, hair clips, toys, and all the necessities she thought little girls needed to be happy. I vividly remember going to a pricey Preparatory school with a lunch bag filled with healthy snacks and fruits and being dressed in fancy stockings and dresses for the school's Christmas pageant and similar events. My dad never failed to provide the finances needed to make provision for the things needed for my survival and wellbeing. He worked very hard as a builder making houses locally and abroad to make this possible. When he was off work and had moments to spend with me, he reminded me that he loved and appreciated me. I believe that a girl who is valued and loved by her dad usually has very high standards in terms of how she allows herself to be treated by others. I could talk to my dad about any imaginable topic. I became a pracademic in the social development field while my dad was a construction worker with a high school education. He appreciated my academic wins, lauded me for them, and encouraged me to carry on.

When my dad died, I landed in a dark place as stepping away from the noise and the limelight to grieve in my closet exposed me to the skeletons I had safely locked away there. On a regular day, I am usually in front of an audience speaking, teaching, or training. Therefore, most times when I am alone, it's time to go to bed or catch up with other duties. Therefore, I was not spending a great deal of time exploring my own feelings. During bereavement, I realised that though I was grieving my dad's death, it seemed there were other unresolved emotions stemming from other trauma throughout my life surfacing for the first time. Dad's death was a moment to pause and to allow myself to "feel." Often, we mask our feelings or try to find worth and fulfilment in things that are inconsequential to our holistic wellbeing. The nakedly vulnerable place I found myself in during the year following my dad's death unmasked me and exposed any charade of confidence I presented. While the theme of my life story is 'from low-self esteem to confidence' and I have been a very confident woman up to the time of Dad's passing, there were noticeable scars from injuries to my self-esteem from which I had not fully healed. During this time, I learnt that for every scar, there was a wound and that sometimes the experience that caused the wound in the first place had such a traumatic impact that the pain does not go away even when the wound closes.

This whole season was a bumpy roller coaster ride as there were days when I had to pull myself together for TV interviews, training sessions or school presentations as I started a Master's degree several months after Dad's passing. After showing up in these spaces, I would nose dive again into the sorrows surfacing from the abusive experiences that kept haunting me. I used this time to delve deep and explore the root cause of trauma I was experiencing.

Navigating grief can be a beautiful journey if you approach it on a quest to find the pockets on your "grief cloak" that carry gifts, life lessons, satisfying joys, new approaches, fresh perspectives, and nutrients to strengthen your mental muscles, just to name a few. I have been on that healing journey. I spent some time in therapy. I spent some time reflecting and researching my trauma responses. I am now enjoying the ebbs and flows of the restorative journey. I have carefully enveloped three approaches in prayer that I am using as my "restoration toolkit."

Emotional Support - Recognizing that I had trauma to deal with and taking the step to do therapy were empowering. I have learnt how to value my own feelings and create boundaries in love. There are many emotional dysfunctions that mask as productive behaviours as they seem to be serving a meaningful cause. For instance, I used to feel validated and valued when I was able to make sacrifices for friends and family members even at the expense of my own well-being. I have learnt that when I am able to maximise my personal well-being, I am much better able to be of optimum benefit to those around me. In the restorative process, I have been setting boundaries and establishing a foundation that keeps me grounded so I do not compromise the mantra that says "caring for my personal wellbeing multiplies my impact on others."

Academic Empowerment - I have also undertaken a journey to understand how the human mind works and what drives our tendencies and responses to situations. In 2012, I completed an undergraduate degree in Psychology that gave me a fairly good understanding of how the mind works. However, the aim on this occasion was to explore what all the knowledge I was garnering meant for me personally. A term I have come to love is the term pracademic, which defines a person whose passion is to apply academic concepts to real life. I have taken this idea from my professional life to apply it to my personal life. As an example, I have spent a considerable amount of time exploring the working of the Reticular Activating System, a part of the brain responsible for how we perceive the world as it regulates our ability to focus and our fight-flight response. In response, I have started focusing on things that will grow my mind and making a conscious attempt to avoid negative thinking triggers. I focus on what I want more of in my life and train my brain to become attracted to these things.

Circle Building - I have realised that after therapy and various types of intervention, certain parts of the healing process have to be done alone. Some internal work is necessary. However, to reinforce all that inner work, it is also important to have a circle around you to provide care, reinforcement, and encouragement. So, I have been intentional about the broader circles in which I operate as these are the spaces we usually attract the people that become closer friends. I have also ensured that the people I draw close to have core values like honesty, authenticity, and genuine care for others as I expect honest feedback when we share situations, feelings, and emotions.

In the process of navigating grief, I have learnt to be more grateful as I learnt the art of scouting all things to be thankful for in a difficult situation. I am grateful to have developed an understanding of the power of intentional healing. I am also grateful that I have been able to develop a deep compassion and insight about other people's feelings. I am able to have a better appreciation for those around me who may show up in certain ways because of trauma. In the deepest parts of my grief, I was stuck in a cycle of repeating self-defeating thoughts. I realised that these thoughts were manifesting negativity in my life and decided to make an intentional effort to break these cycles. I set up accountability systems with friends to cut off negative conversations quickly and redirect energies from negative to positive based on the concept that where energy goes, energy flows. I have learned to love and allow myself to be loved. This has led me to support many people in starting their healing journeys. This includes people who are in my immediate circle who have had a chance to become more beautiful people.

My experiences with grief and trauma have impacted my profession as a Social Development Consultant. The work that I have done with myself as I process personal grief helps me to be better able to recognize when individuals, groups, and communities struggle because of trauma that affects their progress. I am a more thoughtful and compassionate professional who is now conscious about avoiding judgement. People from various communities, whether geographic or social communities, usually act based on the cultures created through their life experiences. Therefore, I approach my work now understanding that the communities I work with understand the anatomy of their needs more than I do and applying my expertise to solve their needs should only come after fully understanding the need from their perspective. When I couple the lessons I have gained from navigating grief, the learnings from the Psychology degree I completed, and the application of principles I have learnt from my mentor, the result is a well-developed character. I have a greater depth of thought and courage to conquer fear and doubt in both personal and professional spheres. Ultimately, I am better able to become stronger because of my grief experience.

When people see those that they look up to as humans with flaws and challenges, it makes the possibility of achieving greatness feel less like an esoteric phenomenon. Simply put, being great feels more reachable. This thought drives my mission to help others grow from the lessons from my mistakes. I have made the mistake of wallowing in my grief and following up with self-defeating actions because I thought my feelings were only valid if someone else validated them. After several years of repeating this behaviour and realising it was robbing my peace, I feverishly searched for an alternative way of behaving. I am now daily building my mental muscles with the understanding that my feelings are valid and it is my responsibility to guard my mental health. I have learnt so many lessons that I now share with the people and I have an opportunity to impact in the spheres of influence to which I have access.

I have gathered the lessons in my R.O.A.R (Retrospective Coherence, Optimism, Antifragility and engaging the Reticular Activation System) toolkit that I share in training and coaching sessions (one-on-one and in groups) across Jamaica in churches, schools, and corporate companies. I also work to empower minorities and disadvantaged communities who have experienced grief in international jurisdictions. For example, I have worked with Black communities in the United Kingdom who lost loved ones during the COVID pandemic using these tools.

Whenever you are facing turmoil, get help to support you to journey through the rough patches and guide you to a place where you can extract the gifts that healing from grief and trauma brings. On the journey of building resilience and becoming antifragile, one often needs a partner to help them navigate through dark moments and discover the silver lining in their clouds.

A better outlook, strengthened mental muscles, and new tools to navigate difficult scenarios easier next time are just a few of the possible gifts from grief.

In Caribbean society, we often overlook some of the manifestations in today's society that are remnants from slavery and colonial rule. This includes the way we show up in our families, the way we parent, the way we manage our organisations, and generally, the way we treat each other. I came to this realisation as I explored the causes of the scars I had. For some of the scars I had, I did not name them or acknowledge prior to my "mental crash." Partner with a therapist, counsellor, or compassionate friend to look at the root of your grief so when you heal, you heal completely and even support other people in your life to heal also.

Steps Towards Intentional Healing

Being intentional about your healing goes beyond cliche statements like "don't worry, it will be fine," and is more about "let's start by writing down the obstacles to overcoming this grief and setting up your navigation plan."

Create a circle of care around you. A circle of care acts as a firm foundation as you navigate grief. Surround yourself with compassionate people who are honest and open to help. Over time, elect some of them to be your partners in overcoming grief and practice with them as you apply new productive habits. For instance, I practice a 30-second rule where I do not allow negative, destructive conversation to continue beyond 30 seconds. My friends cut me off once I reach the limit, and if it is a new story and I want to vent, I must ask for permission and move to a more productive space once I am done venting.

Take breaks. The lessons from our grief takes a certain mindset and time to process the lessons. There is a myth popularised in the 21st century that you must keep going no matter what if you are strong and goal-oriented. This is far from the truth, as one must exercise wisdom and take small breaks to allow your mental muscles to rebuild after distress. It can be so powerful and refreshing when you take a few days to process lessons and make a conscious decision about your new actions. Write down your lessons and write down your new plans after you've done some thinking and processing (retrospective coherence).

Document the lessons and other gifts you have gotten from your trauma. Keep a journal where you make notes about productive ways of being that you've learnt from your grief. Let's call it your "Gifts from Grief" Journal. Include new concepts you've learnt from a counsellor, friend, video, or online research. Also, include new actions you will now take as a result.

Resources

Facebook: Tishaunaindomitablemullings

LinkedIn: Tishaunaindomitablemullings

Instagram: @tishaunaindomitablemullings

CHAPTER 10

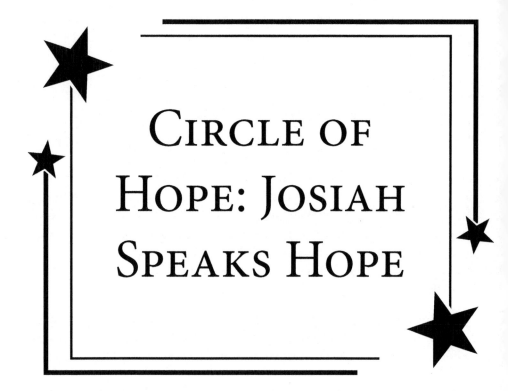

CIRCLE OF HOPE: JOSIAH SPEAKS HOPE

By: LATOYA PINNOCK-WILSON

LATOYA PINNOCK-WILSON

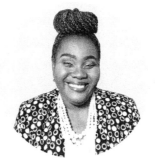

God's promises stand! "There is always a miracle after a loss. Tears turn to testimony, and rejoicing comes after the revelation." - Latoya Pinnock-Wilson (2022)
For I know the plans I have for you, 'Saith the Lord,' they are plans for good and not for disaster, to give you a future and a hope." - Jeremiah 29:11 (NLT)

Pastor Latoya Pinnock-Wilson is a mother, wife, daughter, sister and friend, and most importantly a servant of King Jesus and an overcomer!

For as long as she can remember, she has been a fighter! She's a woman who knows her limits but isn't afraid of surpassing them. She has grown so much over the years and has learned what it means to see the glass as half full rather than half empty. She chose to walk on and to be brave! Holding on to the promises of God and trusting, although it proved to be a hard feat, she pressed on by faith and saw the morning that came after midnight.

She now is an advocate for others who have experienced a loss such as this to help bring hope to those who need not only a shoulder to cry and lean on, but also to help them to navigate through their time of pain and suffering. She helps to lead them to where they can face this season boldly and write their own story in a new light; she offers her services as an ordained pastor, Christian, and mental health/grief counselor, providing hope for those who need it!

INTENTION

It is quite natural for anyone to collapse under the helplessness and the hopelessness that comes with the loss of a child. My hope is that as you read this story you will find hope in knowing that God's promises stand true. It is important to draw on those things that would provide strength, courage, and faith to believe that there will be healing. There will be days to come where you can experience joy and peace and even a miracle!

I want to also convey to my readers that delays are not meant for harm but to build character and develop emotional strength so that by going through such situations with a positive perspective, you will be able to cope and find acceptance through times of grief.

CIRCLE OF HOPE: JOSIAH SPEAKS HOPE

My husband and I attended the same high school; he was a year older, handsome, and quite popular amongst his peers. I was a nerd and he was a deputy monitor for our entire school. We had little to no interaction back then. A few years later after high school, our paths crossed on the Logos Book Ship on a volunteering mission.

Our first date was at the Pegasus Hotel. It was a beautiful first date. We dated for a year and then decided we would take things to the next level. We made the decision to get married! We got engaged, I moved out of my parents house in July, and then we got married in December of 2005.

Life as a young couple was quite good! We were going on dates once every month and were both actively participating in church. Our connection with each other and intimacy with God made our marriage joyous.

My first pregnancy was a miracle and exciting! It was epic to be pregnant with my firstborn in my third year of marriage. We had decided to get pregnant, despite the doctor saying we would not be able to do so! We had a beautiful baby boy, whom we named Joshua after the mighty man of God and leader in the Bible. It was not easy at first being first-time parents, but we made it, balancing ministry, work, and parenting.

Joshua's successful birth strengthened our faith and belief in God to expand our family, but with complication after complication and hormonal issues, we became somewhat disheartened. Nevertheless, we kept trying, kept believing, and declared the Word of God over our lives. In 2018, I received a profound prophetic word that I will conceive a child before the year ends. To be honest, it was a tough word to receive from the woman of God at that moment because of my hormonal issues. My husband and I had started to shift our focus in prayer to give thanks for the prophetic word. We asked God to help our unbelief, and we declared the promises of God constantly! A few months later, I was pregnant!

Now, won't God do it!! Yes, He will. God kept His word.

Twelve years later, we had another miracle boy called Josiah. Sharing this news with my friends and family was a true testimony of God's goodness and that it is with us always! On April 22, 2019, I went for my regular doctor's check-up at the clinic. I was surprised to find that I was 34 weeks pregnant. I also felt really good. Minutes later, I was called in from the waiting room to the assessment room, and as the doctor assessed me, I realized that something felt off about her silence. She was not talking back to me and I became very nervous and concerned.

She stopped and then said, "Mrs. Wilson, I am so sorry but something is not looking right with the baby's heart. It's not beating steadily. We have to rush you off to the hospital." On my way to the hospital, I called my tribe for prayer. My husband and I were anxious and scared, and our emotions were like a roller coaster. We got to the emergency labor and delivery room, and the doctor came to us with the test results and a report for which I certainly wasn't ready. He took a seat and said the words I will never forget. "I am sorry, but we aren't getting a heartbeat from your baby." This was hard to believe and even harder to process. When I asked why I could still feel movements from my baby, he explained that it was just spasms. After hearing that, everything seemed to move in slow motion. It felt unreal. I could hear the doctor as he spoke those painful words. "I'm sorry, there was nothing more we could do." My baby was dead.

I found myself unable to breathe or think properly. It felt like the whole situation was out of my control. I cried so hard! It was as if my heart was ripped out of my chest. I was told by the doctor that they had to do a C-Section to remove the dead baby. This was real. I thought, "This is happening." My baby didn't make it. No, no, no… While I was getting prepared for surgery, I kept praying, hoping, and believing that God would come through for me. That was until they took my baby by C-Section and the long-awaited cries were never heard. My world was shattered…

This experience was an unexpected one. As much as we experienced miracle after miracle, we also met disappointment after disappointment. I learned from early on in this journey that I was going to need faith and dependence and reliance on God. So as much as staying down and wallowing in self-pity seemed easier, I knew that it was going to take work! And it took a lot of stretching and pushing beyond my own strength. I had to show up for counseling, show up at meetings, be there for the difficult times, show up for my family, and most importantly I had to show up for myself.

I doubted, but after spending much time with God and in His word, praying as a family, placing my cares, my pain and my complaints, before God, I gained the strength to start speaking positively about my situation. I started finding things for which to be grateful. I found ways to help others and I learned how to just be honest! I could be honest about how I felt and about how confused and helpless I felt. Giving up was not an option; overcoming was! "Keep pressing on!"

The peer support group I joined is where I received my therapy as an individual and on a group level. I was at a really dark place where depression got the best of me, I was angry all the time, and it was very difficult to parent after the loss of Josiah. I felt very confused and I found myself second-guessing every decision that I made. I was looking for acceptance and validation in everyone and anyone. I felt like a failure to everyone, but most importantly, to my husband and Joshua.

There were days I felt like I was dealing with my grief and others I felt alone as if no one understood what I was going through. I was having so many triggered moments and all the while not knowing how to handle them in a healthy way. Dealing with pain comes with the whole process. I had to be deliberate in making action plans, journaling, and understanding that it was not my fault as I coped and adapted day by day, week by week. I made it a priority to spend time with God, reclaiming my worth in God, not in man. My affirmations and declarations became my strength. Accepting Josiah's death helped me to live again! In July 2021, we had our miracle baby girl, Janiah. She was not a replacement for Josiah. This is just tangible of how God restores peace, hope, and joy to our family and tribe. Janiah is a true example of how God's promise stands no matter our circumstance; just know that it does not matter what it looks like, feels like, smells like, tastes like, sounds, like God is God and He can't change. He is able to do all things well.

Practicing proper breathing exercises and meditating on the Word of God helped massively! I can't stress this enough! I realized from therapy that I can hold a space of happiness and sadness at the same time and that it is all a part of the grief process. There were times I got frustrated and angry with the emotions of missing my son. Compressive, concise, and calming guidance coupled with practical examples and activities helped us, the bereaved parents, in the time when we needed it. The sessions were unique, encouraging, and motivating, touching every aspect of my life and they helped to save me. With compassion, sensitivity, and passion to help others, I myself have experienced this and I have been and will be breaking the silence and taboo surrounding pregnancy loss and infertility issues. I can now facilitate safe space awareness, advocacy, education, and empowerment to all Angel parents.

Through our non-profit organization created in memory of Josiah, my husband and I provide a monthly holistic peer support group meeting, quarterly brunch for Angel Moms, yearly women empowerment conference, an Angel Dads game night, and yearly family retreats. We believe that "Together We Rise," so I salute all our Angel Parents for intentionally healing from scar to stars.

The loss of my son caused overwhelming grief that played out into sadness, regret, anger, and other emotions. I didn't know that I would ever experience that or be a part of that statistic of black women who suffer a stillbirth. Grief peer counseling has offered me lots of ways to handle painful experiences, healthily and holistically. I experienced all stages of grief: denial (this can't be happening to me), anger (I was angry at everyone, even God), bargaining (I wanted my son so badly and it was hard feeling helpless), and acceptance (I started to consider that God must have had a plan for my life). At one point, I felt like it all seemed unfair and I blamed everyone, including myself, but time does heal all wounds!

I had to shift my focus, reframe my way of thinking, and take deliberate actions to be better and healthier! I am grateful for my experience because now I am a proud Angel Mom and I am intentionally healing daily, embracing my scars, and shining on. I can now shine everywhere and at any time for Jesus! I learned how to be diligent in my life duties and in searching the scriptures to know the truth about how much God loves not only me but others. I grew to trust Him more. I became a woman of integrity, I learned how to ask for help whenever I needed it, and I grew closer to my husband and my tribe through it all.

I learned that God is bigger than my battle! I had to stop focusing on the problem and put the focus on my Provider– God! I had to live and be grateful, giving God praise in all things, knowing that everything will ultimately work out for me! God's ways are not man's ways! I know that in life you won't always understand what He's doing, but trust Him. Delay doesn't mean denial! God can move suddenly in your life and cause a shift in everything! I went through a situation that I thought would break me, and that would leave me without hope, but with the help of therapy and those who support me, I can say that the story has progressed to me being much stronger and more hopeful than where I started. I look back, counting it all joy.

From my experience, I became passionate about helping other women who have gone through similar experiences or are currently going through them. My husband and I knew then that we had a calling on our lives, and so we prayed for God's direction. Then the answer came! Our non-profit organization was founded in memory of our son and was named after him, Josiah Speaks Hope, where we speak hope into the lives of women and families, guiding them through their process and their journey. We provide a support group for families and we use a holistic approach for couples that are affected by pregnancy loss and infertility issues among other concerns. We provide a safe space for women to share their stories and make memories.

We also help families to connect with various resources and materials that would assist them with their particular needs. We assist them with coping with the new normal and allowing the couples to acknowledge that they are still parents, even though their baby is deceased. By sitting on the board of the Broward Fetal and Infant Mortality Review Committee, I function as the voice for those who have no voice, allowing their needs be made known. Where there is hope, there is faith; where there is faith, miracles happen.

We all have stories and our story comes with scars; embrace every part of your journey because each scar reminds you of how you have overcome. We're all unique and extraordinary, which makes us stronger, wiser, and more impactful to others and the world at large. Treasure the beautiful memories of your pregnancy and all throughout your journey while your child lived. It won't be easy at first, but you will surely arrive at a place of rest and peace of mind if you stay on the path of healing. You can be brave, courageous, and do the work. And know that you certainly got this! Angel parents, you got this!

STEPS TOWARDS INTENTIONAL HEALING

The most important part of being intentional about your healing is pushing through your pain.

Set realistic goals. Set goals for yourself that will release the stress and pressure that people try to place on you. We all grieve differently so healing looks different for everyone. There are many emotions that come with grief, so journaling, exercising, and meditating are methods of handling triggers and helping monitor and encourage a healthy thought process.

Embrace the importance of having a tribe or village. Healing is a one-day-at-a-time process. Have the right person to pour positive affirmations and encouragement into you, knowing that you have someone by your side to cheer you on every time you accomplish some level of growth in your healing journey. Your tribe will ensure you take care of yourself holistically. They will allow you to be yourself and provide a safe space for you to grow. Your environment plays a great role in who you allow into your space, and what you allow into your spirit can determine how you heal.

Reward and celebrate yourself for your accomplishments. Whether the task that you have accomplished is small or large, you deserve to be rewarded. Applying self-care is very important, and it is vital for you to be gentle, understanding, and compassionate to yourself for any level of healing and growth to take place. When you do accomplish something, reward yourself. Believe in yourself and in the Word of God, which is the blueprint to successful healing as all good and perfect gifts that come from the almighty God belong to us. You are stronger than your pain. Your scars have a story, so share it! Words are powerful, so speak life over yourself. "I am Healed and I am an overcomer." Be your own biggest supporter! Together We Rise!

RESOURCES

Facebook: Josiahspeakshope

Instagram: @Josiahspeakshope

Website: www.josiahspeakshope.org

CHAPTER 11

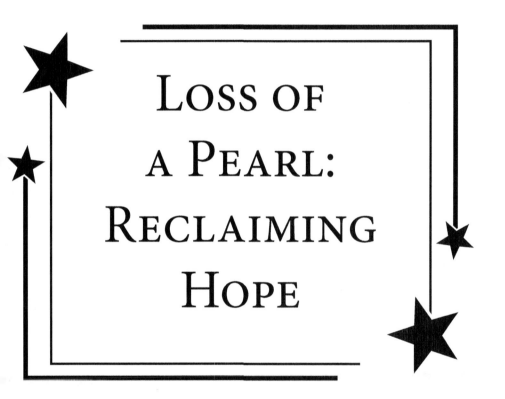

LOSS OF A PEARL: RECLAIMING HOPE

BY: **DR. JOAN M. LATTY**

DR. JOAN M. LATTY

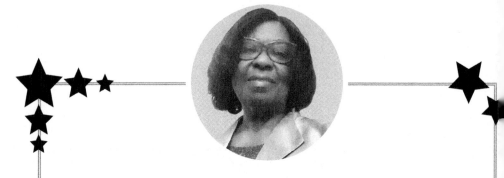

When loss and life's challenges get you down, be renewed by courage, resilience, and Hope. - J. Latty (2022)

Dr. Joan M. Latty is a warm, friendly, fun-loving person who brings light in a dark room, while electrifying the atmosphere with her charm, enthusiasm, and charisma; Jamaican, born in Ewarton, St. Catherine, she is an active devoted SDA Christian. She has been married to her best friend, Joseph, for over 40 years with two adult children, Jaunell and Joseph Junior, two grandchildren, Rojaune and Roger Junior, son-in-law, Roger Miller, and daughter-in-law, Nicole Latty.

She earned a Doctoral Degree in Clinical Psychology from California Southern University, M.Sc. in Counselling Psychology with an emphasis in Marriage and Family Therapy, and a B.A. in Education with a minor in Counselling from Northern Caribbean University (NCU). Joan enjoyed 18 years of teaching at the primary through university levels and over 30 years as a Therapist. She is a Licensed Clinical Psychologist with The Council of Professions Supplementary to Medicine (Jamaica) and The Council for Professions Allied to Medicine, Grand Cayman; she is also a Certified Clinical Supervisor, Ethics Co-Chair, and immediate past Vice President of the Jamaican Psychological Society.

Having previously served as the Director of The Counselling and Psychological Services Centre (CPSC) at NCU, Dr. Latty presently serves as the Clinical Manager and Clinical Psychologist at The Wellness Centre, Cayman Islands. Joan's philosophy is "Let the mind of the Master be the master of my mind as I serve humankind."

INTENTION

I would like readers to know that life is a journey and that death is inevitable. Grief is an expensive commodity with a high cost associated with the loss of someone dearly loved (a pearl). Regardless of the type or magnitude of your scars, there is hope. You can grow through this process towards intentional healing.

LOSS OF A PEARL: RECLAIMING HOPE

As I thought of when life was great, I think of the year 1978 when my darling mother in the bloom of her life at age 45 enacted this sunset scene at the sea. Life was splendid, engorged with beautiful memories of fun, laughter, excitements, fond recollections of good times, family unity, values, playtime, music, and daily devotions. At that time, my immediate family lived in Porus, Manchester, Jamaica. My husband and I taught at the Porus Secondary School. At the beginning of the summer holiday, we decided to take our only child, our two-year-old daughter, to visit my parents in Ewarton.

My husband decided to remain home to finalize business to join us the next day. My daughter and I were on our way. We stopped at my best friend's house in St. Catherine. She was so excited to have us and thought it fun to come along with her young son. All four of us journeyed to my family home in Ewarton, St Catherine. We arrived midday Tuesday. My mother, Ina Benjamin, was just returning from collecting her teacher's salary at Lluidas Vale All Age School. I can still remember her in that beautiful rose-pink dress, which reflected a glow and radiance on her face. From the opposite direction, she beamed with joy, smiled, greeted, lifted her granddaughter, hugged, and kissed her, commenting on how we reached the house at the same time.

We settled down, ate, and talked. While sitting on our favorite seat nestled between and under two large hibiscus trees, mother began trimming my father's hair as she would sometimes do for my four brothers. She said, "Mr. Ben, I have never seen this before. Have you noticed how the guinep and bread-fruit trees have borne? You know, I have heard that when you see this type of special phenomena, it means that someone is going to die."

Later that same evening, we went to church leaving my friend who stayed with my daughter and her son. As we proceeded to leave the house, my youngest brother K, only 10 years old at the time, was having a headache and so he asked my mother to stay with him and not go. She gave him medication and saw to it that he felt better then told him she had to go because she was taking a major part in the crusade. For some reason, my mother did not drive her car that night. We ascended in the back of a pickup van provided by the evangelist to transport the brethren.

Off we went. I was so happy to see the familiar faces after being separated for a long time. I thought to myself, This is the best night I will ever have. The fellowship was grand and service was full of life and enthusiasm. The choir song and sermon were very inspiring and well received. As the service came to a close, the prayer band met. What was revealed to me after was startling and comforting. Mother was the first and only one who prayed, leaving them feeling transported to heaven.

Soon after the dismissal, persons traveling to Ewarton from Crossroads went in the evangelist's van. I looked across at my mother. She smiled at me and said not a word, looking quite pleased. The night was quite still with hardly another vehicle in sight. The night sky shone with beauty and splendor. The clear blue background draped the twinkling stars with a beaming moon. The face of the moon seemed to look down with a stare while the rolling countryside flashed past us. The air was fresh and crisp as the cool breeze caressed our faces. By now, the talking and greeting subsided to whispers. After negotiating our first deep corner, I looked ahead and saw an approaching light. Then suddenly, I heard Bang! Crash! Bang! Screams! Scream! Screams! In a split second, I looked up in the sky while being thrown from the van. I landed on my head. Disoriented and covered in blood, I got up and started to run in the opposite direction from home. I was rescued by a Rasta-man who made every effort to console me. I suddenly remembered that my mother and five of my siblings were in the van. Amid the chaos and the noises of the ambulance screams came the frantic voice of my brother exclaiming, "Thank God! I have found her. J, you okay?" I asked for my mother. They said, "You mean Miss Ben? O she is all right man, but you need to go to the hospital." Whenever I asked for my mother and I was told she was okay. "She is better than you," or, "Oh, Miss Ben has head injuries and will be admitted." When I insisted on seeing her, they said I should go home first as I was not in a position to see her. I asked someone whom I trusted to speak to the doctor and ask for a transfer for her to go to the Spanish Town or Kingston Public Hospital. This was guaranteed. I returned to the car, nervous, terrified, and shaken. In disbelief, shock, and despair, it all felt like a nightmare. I got home at about 3:00 A.M. on Wednesday morning.

I was still curious at the thought that my mother was better than me, yet, I could not see her. Later that morning, I was taken to a private doctor to attend to my oozing head wound. The news was being read on the radio in the doctor's office, which he quickly turned off at the mention of the accident. He immediately started attending to my wound then looked compassionately into my eyes and said, "I am going to sedate you as you are so tired and need a lot of rest." He gave me an injection then bent over and said, "There is something I will have to tell you. You are a big woman now and should be able to come to grips with certain situations, and find ways to handle them."

My heart skipped a beat as the injection started to take effect. I heard his distant wavering voice saying, "Your mother died in the accident last night." I could hear my own voice screaming and in agony, I said, "My mother is not dead; my mother is not dead. No, my mother did not die. She cannot die!" Of course, I kept yelling in denial and disbelief.

As the story unfolded, I learned that my mother had died on the spot. The upcoming weeks were terrible. By Thursday, I was up and about trying to get things in order. Days, weeks, and months passed, and it was now time to physically move on. By now, it was the end of August 1978. I needed to return to my home with my husband and daughter. I needed to return to work in September. I had to break loose and leave my siblings alone with my father, who was still totally devastated and unable to cope.

What must I do? Alas! It was time. I made up my mind to close my eyes and leave for home. The usual jovial, vivacious happy roars of a family of 11, 4 boys, 5 girls, mother, and father, suddenly turned into a bellow of hopelessness and one less. I packed and was on my way out of the house. This experience seemed worse than the death of my mother. All my siblings started crying and pleading with me to stay. They could not survive without me and neither could I survive without them in the absence of our mother. Confused, without the knowledge and consent of my husband, I quieted them down, reassured them, prayed, and decided single-handedly, to unpack and stay. Miraculously, while at church that night, I got a job offer from the principal of the nearby Mt Rosser Primary. Without thinking I simply said, yes. When I got home, I started thinking about what a foolish thing I had done. I still had another job waiting for me, and I had my husband and my child waiting for me; this was crazy. I knew it was crazy but could do nothing about it. When I informed my darling husband, he was so understanding and supportive.

My husband and I developed a visiting relationship for one full year. While being without a helper, I took care of my father, my siblings, and my baby girl. By the end of the school year, 1979, our prayers were answered, and my family was reunited. We both got jobs to teach in Kingston, where we lived and worked for 10 long years.

This traumatic experience impacted me negatively. It was so intense that I never allowed anyone to transport or chauffeur me around. I ceased taking public transportation. To protect myself, I became so overprotective, ensuring that I was kept safe from an accident or anything negative. I was not only protective of myself and my young family but ensured that my siblings and dad were all taken care of as well, even though I think I went overboard.

So how did I navigate my pain, hurt, and loss? I thought it a wise decision to change my environment and relocated to the inner city of Kingston, Jamaica. I had to come to grips with the reality of this loss. Moving made this more bearable. I also changed the focus of my job and I immersed myself in youth work activities that required me to help hurting humanity, Family Life Ministry, guidance counselling, life insurance, always keeping occupied doing something meaningful, especially things that required me helping hurting humanity.

Regardless of how negative this experience has been, it has prepared me for many things in life for which I am now grateful. Without this experience, I would not have been able to go through subsequent experiences with death, in particular the death of my second daughter, my father, my dear sister Rosie and Brother Lloyd. I hold valuable the fact that my husband had not accompanied us and that my friend changed her mind to remain home with my daughter and her son (God's protection on their lives). The seemingly senseless sacrifice of giving up my job, leaving my husband by himself to care for our two-year-old daughter to remain in the family home to support my father and siblings evidently paid off. I am eternally grateful and indebted to my supportive and understanding husband. Instead of continuously mourning the loss of a pearl, I have reclaimed hope, courage, and resilience. I treasure the wonderful legacy that my mom's life has left me. I find myself emulating many of her good qualities while remembering some of the outstanding attributes, values, and behaviors she exemplified. I am grateful that I have become a better person having walked in the footsteps of this phenomenal woman. I now acknowledge that my own experience with grief and managing the resulting trauma might have informed my becoming a Clinical Psychologist with a keen focus in traumatology and helping.

This experience has made me a better person in relation to my understanding of the grief process. My ability to cope increased my sensitivity toward the needs of others experiencing loss and grief. I have become fully aware of the sense of intense emotions (heightened sense of fear, and danger) that accompany grief. This has led to the development of clinical skills as well as a highly supportive and empathetic stance. I am more courageous in journeying with the bereaved and better able to extend care, support, and compassion. I have developed a keen sense of healthier balance between responsibility and accountability to myself, my immediate family and siblings, and by extension my clients.

With a stronger desire to support others during their time of grief, I have become very supportive, not only of my siblings but just about anyone who is going through difficult situations, especially when experiencing grief due to death.

Over time, my focus has evolved into a supportive role in which I attend funerals to intentionally support the bereaved. For me, funerals are solemn events not for frivolity or fun. I do not allow other people to distract me from supporting and being present for the bereaved. I value that moment. Taking care of the bereaved adds an element of care, purpose, and support.

Writing this chapter is the beginning of documenting the legacy of a pearl and reclaiming hope. I will preserve her rich legacy by publishing her life story. My unfinished memoir will also be completed and published so others with similar scars can find one other story to encourage them as they navigate their scars to heal intentionally.

Over the years, I have been and will continue using my hobbies to bless others: singing, organizing, and conducting seminars, workshops, and retreats for couples, empowering and mentoring the youth, promoting mental wellness, and effecting change in the face of loss and societal decline.

We are all aware that life has its ups, downs, twists, and turns. Loss has a way of changing how we function emotionally, physically, socially, and spiritually, throwing us into a state of vulnerability. When all things seem to be going downhill and there seems to be no hope, be assured that HELP is available. Think of life as a university in which we learn how to work through these experiences and how to navigate our scars. Most importantly, determine how to cope and grieve in your own unique way as you should and in your own time. Recall the positive experiences that have happened, the great things you can remember about the individual you loved so dearly, and how you want to commemorate that person's life, especially when they have been influential and have greatly impacted your life. It's not time to fold up; it's time to commemorate all the positive traits and bask in their legacy. My final word of encouragement is to stick to the task at hand, embrace your reality, accept your loss, and move toward your new normal.

Steps Towards Intentional Healing

Here is the HELP you need to effectively navigate your scars and experience Intentionality:

Hold dearly to the memory of your loved one: Effective grieving allows you to be able to embrace your loss, heal, and preserve the memory and legacy of your loved one. One Aeschylus said, "There is no pain so great as the memory of joy in present grief." This was also validated by Marcel Proust, who said, "Happiness is beneficial for the body, but it is grief that develops the powers of the mind."

Educate yourself: Everyone, at some point in his or her life, will experience loss; it is important that you seek to educate yourself about the benefits of appropriate grieving. Education helps you develop your internal locus of control, improve your emotional regulation, and build resilience to navigate the grieving space.

Life - Have a balanced life: Grief has a great impact depending on attachment and how the person died, creating a level of vulnerability, chaos, and imbalance, however people get to a place of acceptance about their loss eventually. This is when you come to grips with the reality that you have to live without the deceased. Grief is an ongoing process but varies from person to person based on a range of factors. It does not mean that you are over the loss, but it means that it is time to create balance. To balance your life, you must come to terms with your loss. Take a break from grief at times and focus on your wellbeing, change your focus from the loss, and deal with your emotions. Practice daily coping and adjust to taking care of your life, learn new ways to live without the loved one, adjust to the changes, and commit to accommodating your new normal.

Positive Emotions: Is it possible to have a positive emotion when there is deep loss, sadness, and pain? Yes. A positive emotion contributes to a person's well-being, and is needed in creating balance in life. During grief, individuals may have a negative view of life; however, positive emotions can be increased by assessing if your current outlook is excessively negative. Give yourself permission to feel positive emotions and identify your source of hope, courage, and optimism. Finally, stay away from negative people, improve your cognitive functioning, and practice and maintain positive emotions. Pray to increase your faith in God and have hope in a positive search for a successful life. HELP is available.

CHAPTER 12

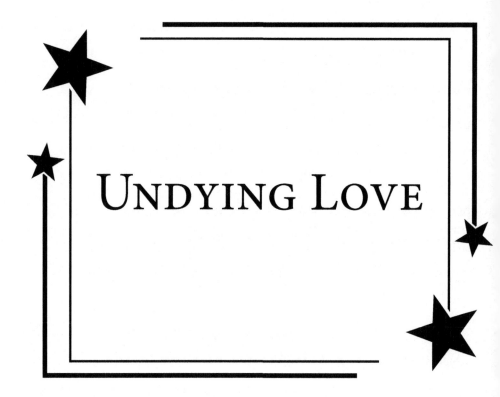

UNDYING LOVE

BY: DR. JUDITH McGHIE

Dr. Judith McGhie

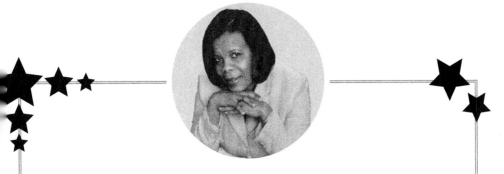

The Lord is close to the brokenhearted and saves those who are crushed in spirit. - Psalm 34:18
"Mother's love is undying and incomparable – in her eyes, you see the purest form of love – she's the one who can take the place of others, but whose place no one else can take." - Samuel P.G. Pryce

Dr. Judith I. McGhie holds a doctorate in clinical psychology and works at a prominent Pennsylvania mental health facility in the forensic department. A native of Jamaica, Dr. McGhie's career spans almost two decades which includes working previously within the prison system in the states of New Jersey and Pennsylvania as a clinician. Her areas of expertise cover community health, persons affected by homelessness, and those who are severely mentally ill. Additionally, she specializes in cases dealing with patients diagnosed with schizophrenia and intellectual delay. She has been the recipient of the Montgomery County Award for outstanding service in the field of mental health and is known to approach her daily tasks with passion, commitment, and professionalism. Prior to her current vocation, Judith was a high school teacher in Jamaica and Saint Lucia; she also served as director of residence halls at university and academy levels in Jamaica and Pennsylvania. In her spare time, Dr. McGhie enjoys traveling, floral arranging, event planning, interior design, sewing, culinary arts, and singing. She is an admitted track and field athletics enthusiast, lover of Colonial Revival homes, and one who espouses Christian principles and values. Judith currently resides in the Commonwealth of Pennsylvania.

INTENTION

It is my sincere wish and desire that my personal account will somehow stir introspection, inspiration and restoration. Experiencing the various stages of grief is difficult and may seem to be an insurmountable task to navigate; however, it is possible. Indeed there is hope and triumph to be derived. I would like for the prospective reader to realize that in spite of feeling heartbroken, vulnerable, and helpless, one does not have to remain in that situation indefinitely. With self-determination, inner resolve, and spiritual fortitude, tragedy will be replaced with triumph. Ultimately, life will take on fresh new meaning.

UNDYING LOVE

Reflecting on memories of growing up in Maroon Town, Jamaica, my philosophy of kindness, empathy, and caring stemmed from the warmth within the home. The importance of etiquette and grooming, the transforming power and value of the family, and the courage to be myself were all introduced and shaped by my incredible mother, Isolyn Gracey Harris. She knew me from my first breath. Mother was beautiful, and she emanated radiance within and without. Life poured from her; she was God-fearing and exuded a Christ-like character.

I tried to emulate her character and soon discovered as I grew older that some of my innate traits came naturally from her, my earthly icon. My mother's focus was not on physical beauty; she would admonish me to "be the best at what you can be, and whatever you do, do it to the best of your ability." Notions of beauty are wide-ranging. I believe my mother's definition of beauty was a combination of moral, spiritual, and intellectual qualities. Though strict, she showed love and nurtured and demonstrated a calming disposition when she corrected me and my siblings. Without uttering a word, she would gaze into our eyes indicating a particular "look" whenever we acted contrary to her expectations. This has taught me to pay rapt attention especially during formal settings.

Being a disciplinarian did not preclude mother from possessing a capricious, humorous, and good-natured spirit. She never said anything to dampen my spirit, thus I have always maintained high self-esteem. My mother was the epitome of grace and dignity. She rarely got upset and I have never heard her raise her voice in discontent with anyone. Soft-spoken yet firm when the need arose, she believed in respect and discipline.

She loved flora, enjoyed gardening, sewing, embroidery, singing, and remarkably learned the art of shoemaking from her father! My mother believed in healthy living, and her cooking and baking skills were legendary. God was her constant companion, as she took everything to Him in prayer. Her reverence for the Lord was so deep that she always covered her head during the act of supplication. Mother was fervent in the study of the Bible. She never missed church services unless it was inevitable. Whenever in despair, my mother's soothing voice was all I needed to restore inner calm. Her words of wisdom continue to govern my life.

I remember leaving the confines of home and my dear mother behind to attend college. This was my first time being separated from her for a prolonged period. A strange feeling engulfed me as I contemplated being away from the "angel" who brought me into this world; the mere thought of not hearing her voice, experiencing a tender touch, and relishing the lovingly prepared meals on a daily basis was unimaginable! I became very emotional and cried every night for several months as this was a new experience for me.

Time went by and many years had passed. I vividly remember the date – it was a spring day, Friday, May 9, 2014. While driving along the highway on my way to work, an unusual and unexplainable sensation enveloped me, a sense of foreboding. It was around that same time that my best friend, my beloved mother, closed her eyes for the last time, although I had not yet learned of her death. Later that evening was when the unexpected news was broken to me. I had intended on traveling to Jamaica to see her that very weekend on which Mother's Day fell; however, the plans did not materialize. Feeling utterly heartbroken, a part of me died that day as a numbness swept over my soul like a tidal wave.

I was in total grief and a mournful state right until the day of the funeral services for my precious departed mother. I was inconsolable and wept uncontrollably, going through the motions and oblivious to the proceedings. A close friend remarked that I wailed the enter time with every fiber within my being. Everything going on around me was like a perpetual blur, and the atmosphere was so surreal. At the interment, a feeling of desolation came over me as if falling into an abyss. I did not stand and watch as she was gently lowered to her final resting place, but rather sat some distance away. It was too much to bear.

My mother is unforgettable, thinking of her constantly comes so easily. Though eight years have elapsed, fresh memories remain in my consciousness. Upon reflection, some days are beautiful and tranquil while others are painful and difficult. Many times I wish it were possible to cuddle within her loving arms to experience that inimitable, penetrating gaze and warm smile. Deep within my heart, she always has a special place.

Over the years since my mother died, my life has changed in various ways and taken off on a trajectory that I would not have foreseen or expected. I have developed and blossomed more and had a greater appreciation for life, living and enjoying each day fully without delaying things until some other time which may not come.

My spirituality has become more enriched, as I have drawn closer to God, and my prayer life has greatly improved. I exercise more faith and have had my prayers answered on numerous occasions. Relying more and more on divine guidance propels me daily. I have grown more resilient to the challenges and setbacks that would present a deterrent to the aspirations and goals I set for myself.

An area that I have delved into is extending myself to helping others in meaningful ways. This includes praying for individuals experiencing a range of issues, including the loss of a loved one or job, loneliness, the stress of elder care, and health issues. One serious issue I dealt with was a friend contemplating suicide. Somehow, after being made aware of the situation, I got involved and providentially a potentially tragic and unfortunate outcome was averted. It brings a sense of satisfaction in helping others to make informed decisions and choices that will improve their lives.

I have become more involved in the sharing of my gifts and talents. What brings me fulfillment is undertaking a project and seeing its execution to the satisfaction of those it was intended. Some areas I have undertaken are emceeing at events, planning weddings for friends, organizing church functions, and preparing and giving presentations with an emphasis on mental health.

Traveling is an outlet that helps in bringing balance to my life and has been of great benefit in the restorative process. Visiting and seeing places away from home contribute to mental well-being and inner calm. It is always delightful and heartening spending quality time and bonding with close friends and family members which ultimately brings feelings of rejuvenation.

I have turned to writing as a part of the healing process, allowing my thoughts to flow and expressing them as they come to mind; poetry and personal quotes from the heart bring peace and comfort. At other times reflecting and reminiscing brings a smile to my face when I consider the pleasant memories which I hold dear.

Mother always encouraged and motivated me from early childhood and was influential in shaping my life's direction. Sometimes I wish she were here to see my progress and for me to dote on her. Thinking of her often has helped me to excel in my career and strive to be goal-oriented. I impart life skills to persons in need of assistance and share knowledge gleaned from my formal studies with others.

As time went by, I became aware of my sensory absorption and surroundings affected my mental state. If I was grief-stricken, depressed or hurt, this could have a negative impact on my personal feelings, so I made a conscious decision to embrace self-care. Realizing that a healthy mind and body makes for a pleasant place to inhabit has proven enabling. I have always been an avid reader and have indulged more in recent times. Getting a spa treatment has proven to be therapeutic and energizing. Decorating and rearranging my bedroom brings about a satisfying feeling too. I believe that making minute yet significant changes in one's life helps to create ascending steps. Being hopeful, positive, expectant and cheerful are attributes that will play a major part in overcoming cataclysmic anguish and dispelling the dark clouds of pain.

My mother's death brought untold anguish and grief. I have come a long way to this present stage. It is said that time brings healing. Structuring and filling each day with meaningful and positive moments has helped me to dispel thoughts of sadness and pain. Each day I strive to develop a positive thought from the many memories I have of her. Having a strong support base is crucial after losing a loved one; I am most grateful for my older siblings, Patsy, Norma, and Ewart, though experiencing grief manifested unconditional love and expressed comfort. They were available to listen and encourage me. My relationship with God has been strengthened. I call on Him for strength and fortitude daily to meet life's vicissitudes.

I am thankful for the Christian values that my mother instilled in me. Each day is valuable and celebrated because tomorrow is not guaranteed. Every morning upon waking, I practice self-affirmation. "I am wonderfully made, I am resilient, I am beautiful," were only a few.

My gratitude for those with whom I live and work the closest propels my responsibility to be enthused and of a pure mind. The impact of the good we do with an open, glad heart and a smile is incalculable.

My mother played a major role in my character-development. Her life of quiet dignity and the Christian-principles she upheld and exhibited had an indelible impact on me. The person I am today is as a result of the life she lived and noble qualities she constantly exemplified. Today, I can be an example to others seeking to self-actualize and be better persons. I am eternally thankful for such a wonderful lady.

My spiritual growth and by extension, my relationship with God, have been contributing factors. Through the mediums of prayer, meditation, and reading the Bible, I have gained strength to face each day feeling fortified. Awaking with an attitude of gratitude and a positive spirit is what sustains me throughout each day. I have acquired qualities of boldness, self-confidence, and assertiveness implemented in various situations whenever necessary.

Another aspect in the development journey is having a passion for sharing my gifts and talents with others. It is always a joy to derive satisfaction from making a positive impact in someone else's life. Receiving an appreciative smile or a word of thankfulness is always heartwarming. I do believe in the act of service and living not for myself only but for others.

I have gradually become more emboldened and revitalized over the past eight years since embarking on my journey "from scars to stars." Challenges and setbacks do not daunt me; instead I draw on inner resolve to face and overcome the hurdles and difficulties that come my way. This is a result of my spiritual maturity and reflecting on my mother. In my quiet moments, I "hear" her soothing voice whispering words of encouragement and motivation.

At least two incidents have occurred fairly recently which have left me pleasantly surprised. Upon entering two business places, an attendant instantly started to smile and shower me with words of admiration and adoration! I can only conclude that there was an aura that caught their attention and drew me to them. These have been touching experiences that have given me the satisfying feeling that I had made someone's day.

I endeavor to portray a positive attitude and cheerful demeanor always. Colleagues at work notice my disposition and remark favorably. Hopefully this will make a meaningful impression and create an avenue they will be inclined to follow.

Losing a loved one is an agonizing and impactful experience. Don't be hard on yourself; take your time to go through the process of grieving, no matter how long it takes, whether months or years. It is important to take care of yourself; do not neglect eating and sleeping. Seek the support of others; this assists in coping and finding solace. Endeavor not to lock yourself away and get depressed; you may be surprised that there are folks willing and able to be there for you without you having to seek them out. Take time out to engage in activities that will divert your mind from feelings of sadness – it may be going for a walk, spending time with a friend who is humorous, or re-engaging in a hobby. Decide how you will fill the hours of each day and have a schedule for each day.

STEPS TOWARDS INTENTIONAL HEALING

1. Seek emotional support, which enhances healing.

2. Develop your faith in God and continue to grow spiritually.

3. Put your thoughts into writing. I have included an example below of a poem I wrote titled "Mother."

MOTHER

We cannot forget the tenderness in our mother's gentle touch.

Her hands were delicately made to soothe our pains that often hurt so much.

We could not overlook the sunshine in her luminous and generous smiles.

Mother showed her love in everything she did to make our lives worthwhile.

Her laughter was a source of joy; her words were warm and wise.

Her loving voice echoed far and near, but never in disguise.

We might not often stop to think of the many things that she gladly did

to bring a little happiness to others throughout the years.

She shared, she cared, she gave, and she listened.

There was such kindness and compassion that we found in her strong embrace.

Just being in her presence, our lives were always filled with goodness and grace.

Mother had a God-given talent to pray for the big and the small,

She would pray to God in earnest, believing He answers all.

Thus, we will forever believe that her praying hands and her Christ-centered heart helped to comfort our troubled hearts.

Thank God for blessing us with a mother who was so loving and so dear,

By looking in her tender eyes we found hope, courage, and good cheer.

God, thank you for our mother, the gift that you gave us

that perfectly fits the size of our open hearts.

We will forever remember our mother with such fondness, love, and care.

And when we think of the wonderful times that we shared

We will hold on to some warm and wonderful memories that we will cherish year after year.   **-Dr. Judith I. McGhie** ©

CHAPTER 13

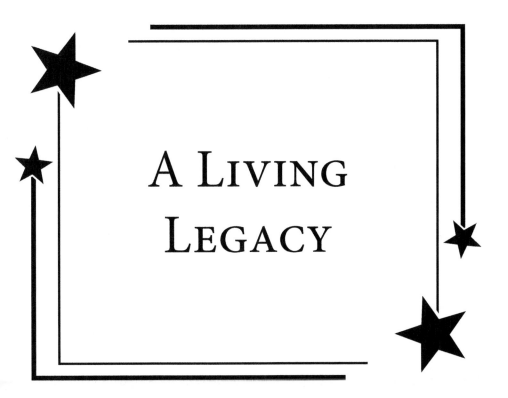

A LIVING
LEGACY

BY: ANDREA FRANCIS

ANDREA FRANCIS

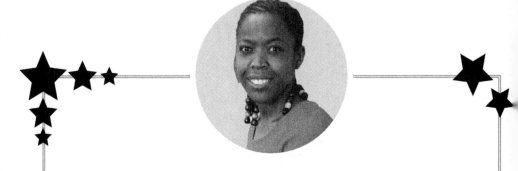

The true measure of your worth is the impact you have after you're gone. - Andrea Francis (2022)

Andrea Francis views herself as God's child and Jennifer's daughter. A diamond shaped in the bowels of life's challenges, the crucibles of disappointment and grief have fashioned her into the woman she is today. An educator by profession, she proudly declares herself the eternal student. She is a preacher, motivational speaker, and youth enthusiast that has the mission of empowering young people to actualize their God-given potential. Learning results in a change in behavior, so as she teaches and learns, she encourages others to do the same while she constantly morphs as she grows while seeking to impact others. God's promises are real and true. She has found "I am with you always" (Matthew 28:20, KJV) to be the best life jacket in the middle of a crisis. She is thankful that He continues to keep His promise as stated in Psalm 27:10, as He is the God who mothers her. This chapter is the latest installment in the writing legacy that Andrea is creating. As Jennifer's legacy, she is a tattered garment in the hands of the Master Designer whose work of fashioning her is ongoing so that she can be fitted for eternity.

INTENTION

When faced with life's challenges, sometimes in a split second you have to decide if you are going to fold under the pressure or press through despite the adversities. Journey through my eyes and see how this choice determines if you successfully weather grief's storm or remain trapped in its bowels. I hope you will learn that you do not need to sink in despair but can rise above your adverse circumstances and find hope, a new sense of purpose, and freedom. Terrible things may happen in life but with intentional work, you can ensure that you have joy in the journey.

A LIVING LEGACY

The sound of laughter echoed in the house as the sisters played together. Mother worked close to them to ensure that they were safe while enjoying themselves. Wafts of food circulated in the atmosphere, giving hints that it was almost time for dinner. Such was a typical afternoon in our household back then. During the week, my older sister and I would get dressed for school which often meant taking pictures on the patch of grass that was the 'lawn' before we departed. On Friday evenings, we had vespers with our grandparents. Grandpa Francis ensured that we had a strong spiritual foundation. We did not know it then but in time to come, that would be a source of strength. But us girls loved Sundays because Daddy was not just more available but prepared dinner. Time had taught us that there was more fried chicken when Daddy cooked. We would eat together and then spend the rest of the evening in each other's company. Life was great then.

I couldn't tell you what age I was when my parents separated. One day I just realized that the well-oiled machinery that was our family had changed. Dad moved to the city, and we stayed with Mom. Thus began our unique living conditions as my sisters and I lived with our mom among my father's family. Adulthood would teach me how rare such a symbiotic family relationship was. Our circumstances were different, but life was good. Mom's life was dedicated to doing what was necessary to rear her three girls properly. Though not physically living with us, Dad remained in our lives albeit in a different portfolio. Growing up in a rural community in St. Thomas, Jamaica, my life revolved around my family, friends, and church community.

The warmth of the sunshine and whisper of the wind in the trees that were all around us, rolling hills, bubbling streams, and grass-covered fields meant we were constantly surrounded by nature. The passage of time resulted in well-defined chores and roles to ensure the efficient running of our household. Mom was a seamstress and would spend countless hours cutting and sewing as she contributed to our financial stability. My sisters and I developed under her watch. The fact that she worked from home meant that she was there when we went out and came in, a constant fixture ready to support and also hold us accountable.

Life settled into a predictable pattern with Mom being the axis around which we rotated. Then one day she became ill. She was hospitalized with a collapsed lung and a diagnosis of pneumonia. But we weathered the storm and she eventually returned home. When she was hospitalized again, I thought we had beaten the illness the last time. With my older sister in the United States, hospital trips became my responsibility.

Each day I commuted by bus and taxi to see her. Mom was a mere shadow of herself. My heart ached as she was apologetic when I assisted with basic toiletries. Imagine my source of support apologizing because I had to complete a few tasks for her. The hospital stay took a toll on her mentally and emotionally. The tests were plenteous until her system said no more as her skin refused to be stuck by another needle. School resumed and as soon as it was out, I headed to the hospital to find that my mom, who could hardly move, had been discharged. Still, we were happy she was home. Over the next few days, she seemed to regain strength and even started to do small tasks. We all thought she was on the road to recovery.

September 18, 1995, is forever etched in my memory. I fixed a meal of stewed chicken and produce for breakfast. I hurried out the door with promises to be home by 6:00 P.M. That day I wanted to skip my evening class but acceded to my friends and stayed. Getting on a bus was a trying task. It would be 7:30 P.M. before I arrived at the town square in the middle of a power outage. "Miss Jennifer dead," my cousin remarked when he saw me. "You too lie!" automatically slipped from my lips but the look on my sister's and relatives' faces confirmed my worst nightmare was true. The half-mile trek felt like two as we walked home in the darkness. I stared at her now unseeing eyes as my heart broke to hear that at ten minutes to six, she said I can wait no longer and breathed her last breath. Mom had been trying to wait until 6:00 P.M., which was the time I had told her I would be back when I left that morning. As my hands slid over her face, her eyes closed easily. Broken, dazed, and just numb, I stood there by her bedside.

I lost count of the number of times I was physically removed from my mom's bedside before the undertakers arrived. I oscillated between being at her bedside and sitting outside playing with my dog. My mind had recollections of past conversations with Mom on repeat. Mom must have had a sixth sense about dying early, I thought as I recalled her encouraging my sisters and me to acquire skills from her before it was too late to do so. Well, now it was officially too late. The only thing I could do is try to fulfill another request, that of us taking care of each other. As the hearse drove on the darkened road away from our house, I felt like a part of me had departed with it. To say that I was numb does not begin to scratch the surface of the loneliness and despair that inhabited my being.

In hindsight, it is interesting how God orchestrates circumstances in our lives. We settled into a new normal as another transition was experienced. We started living with Dad in the same home we used to live with Mom. Dad hovered close to me and my younger sister. In the days after Mom's death, our house was a buzz with people coming and going. Despite the flow of people, there was this void that no one could fill. And then, how could they? How could they fill the gap created by the woman who was the center of my world? Days blurred together as I traversed life A.M. – after mom. The weather seemed to concur with the turbulent situation that was my life. One bleak, rainy day morphed into another. On the day of her funeral, it rained copious showers that were the tears I found myself unable to cry. Perhaps because I had always told my mom I would not.

Intentional Healing: From Scars to Stars

The effervescence with which I approached life became methodical as I developed a routine for going through the days. Busy became my sanctuary, once I was busy I would not have to process my thoughts and emotions. I could get by and make it through each day. But God made sure that I was reminded that He had not forgotten me. I will not tell you that it was easy because it was not. He ensured that there were more people that cared for me than those who saw Mom's death as the opportune time to advance their personal agendas. Four years and three months after her death, I finally cried. As I listened to another daughter relating her mom's death, I saw myself in her story and cried. I cried for my mom's death, for what could have been and never would be, for what was and would no longer be. After that God started leading me on a road to recovery, a path where I would cherish each memory of the life I lived with my mother and work to actualize the woman she envisioned I would become. I would make that woman a reality so that even though my mother was dead, her dreams would last beyond her lifetime. Throughout that journey, God has been a constant. He proved His word true over and over again. When I missed lying across my mom, He was there and held me in His arms or provided a surrogate mother for me to lay across. He keeps providing mentors that fill the gap and provide nurture and motherly care. I am eternally grateful for my 'Mother God' who keeps mothering me and ensures that I am not motherless.

There is a grave danger of falling prey to becoming entangled by the cruel beasts called despair, self-pity, and guilt. However, after God helped me to crawl through the tunnel of despair and cross the chasm of guilt, I found a lot to be grateful for and came to the realization that God was making me stronger. I benefited from the nurture of a phenomenal woman who taught me the value of kindness, humility, and industry. She had poured selflessly into not just the life of my sisters and me but several individuals. Almost thirty years after her passing, she is fondly remembered, and not just by family members. I aspire to have such a legacy and be a transformative agent. I am grateful that God has never left me and continues to place persons in my life that are sources of encouragement and blessings. I am not a victim; I am a victor who has weathered the storms of grief and disappointment and emerged stronger because of my experiences. God has created an oasis where there once stood a desert. That is something I can share with others in similar circumstances.

I am coming to the realization that Isaiah had in Isaiah 6 when king Uzziah died. Mom was my rock. If that rock was never moved, I would have failed to truly see the Rock of Ages who has become the foundation upon which I stand. I wish I could tell you that I could say that there was a groundbreaking moment when I suddenly comprehended that there was value in my brokenness. God is still actively working on me, building resilience, depth of character, and a thirst to empower others. Truth be told, at times I have hindered His work and He had to replace a sleeve or stitch a hem here and there. The garment is still being fashioned and my story continues to be woven. The journey has taught me that I have nothing to fear. The numb girl has become a not-so-numb adult who has learned that the users, the abusers, and opportunists are nowhere as important as the nurturers, supporters, and surrogates that God has blessed me with. My glass is totally filled, and God has used all my life's circumstances to shape my character to make me a better person and a stronger Christian.

Rising above the numbing impact of losing my mother took deliberate effort. This was not a work that was done in my own strength but through God's enabling. As I was bogged down by the intensity of my grief, God led me through a proverbial exodus from the doldrums of despair. During these moments, I clung tightly to Phillipians 4:13 (KJV), which says, "I can do all things through Christ," and it became a mantra for me, much more than a Bible verse I had memorized as a child. I was better able to not just fully live but also encourage others as they journeyed through their grief. My challenge became a ministry platform as I counsel countless individuals about pressing through their grief and being able to live again. The true measure of your worth is the impact you have after you're gone. My mother left a lasting impact on me and her legacy lives on through the life that I live. My mission is not only to impact others by how I live my life but to empower them to join me on the journey to building living legacies that will influence the lives of others for years to come.

The butterfly does not become a beauty overnight. As a caterpillar, it spends its days eating leaves and storing energy for when it will be needed. The chrysalis is suspended in time and space until nature tells it the time is right to break free from its cocoon. When it does, it's perfectly formed and ready to fly. Grief is crippling and debilitating but victory lies in acknowledging and treating it. Your experiences will fuel your transition.

It is time to break free of its shackles and join other butterflies who have encountered similar yet distinct journeys. Together let us fly from plant to plant sipping nectar while positively contributing to the ecosystem as a pollinator making life better for other organisms. Use what you have learned from wading through your scars for the empowerment of others as you become the star that illuminates their path.

Steps Towards Intentional Healing

As you seek to heal intentionally and build a lasting legacy, here is a TIP that you can follow:

Treasure the memories of wonderful moments that you spent together as a family. Remember them with joy so they can wash over you like the cleansing power of a waterfall that invigorates as it hits your skin. Celebrate the moments you shared which are testaments of a life well lived. As you practice this, you will find that you will no longer focus on your loss but instead will see all that you have been left with as a legacy.

Inhabit the present and embrace new experiences. Yield not to the temptation of living in the past. There will be an abundance of both good and bad moments but know that your loved one would want you totally free from the deadly grasp of 'could haves' and 'should haves.' Fully embrace life and create new experiences. Your grief will not suddenly disappear, but you will find that you would have carved a path that leads you through your grief. This is not an impossible task; with God's help you, too, can make it because I did.

Practice gratitude. Being grateful each day will keep you grounded, especially in those times when you feel that you have a tenuous hold on who you are as a person and the purposefulness of your existence. The more you find to be grateful for, the more meaningful your life will become. Too often we focus on all that is awry and miss the wonder of all that is wonderful. Purpose to focus on the good, even if you have to search for it with a magnifying glass.

Resources

Linktree: https://linktr.ee/jenlegacywrite

Linkedin: https://linkedin.com/in/andrea-francis-b0897477

CHAPTER 14

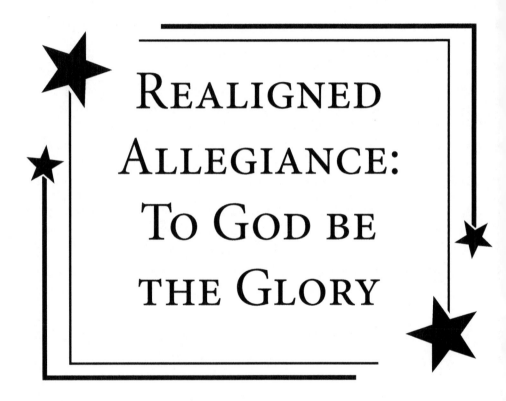

REALIGNED ALLEGIANCE: TO GOD BE THE GLORY

BY: CHAUNA-KAYE POTTINGER

CHAUNA-KAYE POTTINGER

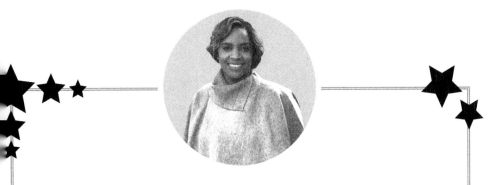

Pursue healing not regret.
- Chauna-Kaye Pottinger (2022)

Chauna-Kaye Pottinger is a motivated, personable, innovative, and outside-of-the-box thought-leader who is undaunted by failure. She lives and breathes her life's calling of uniting her God-given skills and expertise with the power of the Holy Spirit to contribute positively to the growth and development of the gospel ministry.

A native of the beautiful island of Jamaica, Chauna-Kaye is married to Jaymie Pottinger. From this union, they have been blessed with three children: JeChaun, Jenna-Peyton, and Jaymie II.

In 2007, she obtained a Bachelor of Science Degree in the field of Management at Northern Caribbean University. She also holds a Master of Science Degree in Project Management from Walden University.

In 2019, she partnered with her husband Jaymie Pottinger and founded a Human Resource Consulting Firm named Pottinger and Associates Consulting. It is a company that helps organizations to align their people strategy with their business strategy to maximize their business results.

In her spare time, she enjoys blogging, doing crochet, and painting. Her greatest hope and ambition is to make it to Heaven and to convince as many people as she can to do the same.

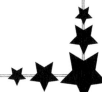

INTENTION

The boulders of adversity and pain placed in our path, which were meant to block our path, when surmounted, will only give us an elevated perspective on the road ahead.

What does a young vivacious, goal-oriented 21-year-old college graduate do when she is faced with tremendous loss and crucibles all within the space of a few months? The shock and pain of losing a mother is preceded by a number of monumentally unfortunate events. Does she spiral out of control, losing sight of her relationship with God? What does she do when the only source of her spiritual connection is pre-maturely severed? All it took was one miracle and a God who loved her enough to show up just when she needed Him most! Through it all, she is sustained and now she shares this story of hope and triumph to anyone who wishes to be inspired.

REALIGNED ALLEGIANCE: TO GOD BE THE GLORY

It was the fall of 2006 and I had just recently decided to travel between Mandeville and St Ann in Jamaica, a two-and-a-half-hour journey each way, to remain on track for graduation in the summer of 2007. For the most part, everything seemed to have been going well. My plan was to take no more than the allotted four years to complete my undergraduate degree and regardless of the obstacles faced, I was fixated on achieving this goal. Though I was young at the time, I observed carefully the challenges my other siblings encountered in college where finances were concerned, and I formulated a plan that I believed would have surmounted many of the challenges they faced.

On my first day of school, I was given a bulletin along with my orientation packet. In one presentation, one presenter used the word "contract" to describe this bulletin. In fact, it was the most important document I received that day and I should guard it with my life. This meant that if we've fulfilled all the requirements outlined in the bulletin, the university is duty-bound to confer upon us the degree commensurate with such requirements. I took this literally. Throughout my tenure at college, the days that I did not take my bulletin along with me to school were few and far between. Its pages were decorated with annotations, dog-ears, and highlighters; it endured the rigors of spilled juices and gravy from my lunch and the ever-popular accidental rips that occurred every now and again as I was reading it while walking.

This bulletin helped to keep me on track. I kept my goals simple and to the point. Goal number one: finish my Associate Degree in Business Administration and graduate in the summer of 2005. Goal number two: get a fulltime job, and attend school on a part-time basis to finish my Bachelor's degree by the summer of 2007. I succeeded with my first goal and the second goal was fulfilled in the fall of 2005.

I landed the right job. A Customer Care Officer position at a government agency was just what I needed. I was a great Customer Care Officer, action-oriented, solution-driven, risk-tolerant, and undaunted by failure. I was ready for the world of work and I was on track to graduate August 2007. Everything was going well with me even though my prayer life was pretty non-existent. After all, I had Mama. I called her when I needed divine intervention, when my boss was giving me a tough time, my professors were being unreasonable, or when Jaymie and I had an argument that warranted prayer. Life was amazing.

2007 was the year from hell. On January 12, I set out on my usual journey from Mandeville headed towards St Ann's Bay. I left thirty minutes earlier than my regularly scheduled departure hoping that I would have a 30-minute head start to my day. Little did I know that this trip would have resulted in my very first car accident. This car accident would have left me with a whiplash and concussion, the pain from which haunts me to this very day.

In the spring, my then boyfriend Jaymie visited from the US and proposed to me on my birthday and I said yes. I was beyond ecstatic to receive his proposal, but within a few short days, I discovered that I was pregnant with my first child. Instead of being overjoyed, I felt shame from letting my mother and God down (in that order). I felt shame from knowing I will have to wear the visible signs of my sinful actions in full view of some church members who were just waiting for something like this to happen.

In June, as I sat in my Marketing Management class doing a test, my brother France came to the door and whispered, "Mama is in the hospital." I fell apart. I had spent the weekend with her and it was very clear that she was not in the best shape, but I never anticipated hospitalization. There I was pregnant, afraid, and ashamed, but now horror-stricken because Mama is not supposed to ever be sick enough to be hospitalized.

A surge of pain ran through the bottom of my belly, my knees felt like jello, and my hands could no longer firmly grip my pen. I gave out a wail that would send off a clear signal that someone was dead. It was almost as if I could sense it. At this point, my non-existent prayer life had now become an intermittent cry to Jesus for his intervention on my mother's behalf. Mama's illness was complicated, but we were all in denial about death being a possibility. Her most serious illness impacted her heart and the other illnesses she had developed from being in the hospital with limited mobility.

On numerous occasions, when her situation worsened, we would send out an alert to our prayer warriors and something miraculous would happen that would make us all think that she was going to be healed. One such miracle was when she became well enough to be released from the hospital in time to witness the graduation of my brother France and me.

Two weeks after her initial release from the hospital, Mama was hospitalized again and without saying goodbye, on October 1, 2007 (four weeks after being hospitalized), Mama succumbed to her illnesses. All the signs pointed to it, but we were too hopeful that the true miracle would come in the form of her healing. What in the world was happening to me? My world was spiraling out of control and turned upside down. There I was in the seventh month of my pregnancy and Mama was dead. She did not even get the chance to enjoy the fruits of her labor after witnessing her last child walk across the graduation stage.

In the weeks that followed, my siblings and I along with our aunts and uncles struggled but succeeded in making the necessary arrangements for Mama's funeral. I cannot find words to describe how terrible it felt. The two weeks prior to her burial were by far the worst two weeks of my life. Maybe the sun was shining at some point during that period, but those were some of the darkest days I've ever seen for a sustained period. Everything seemed gray. The pain I felt was as physiological as it was emotional. There was a gaping hole in my chest. Why Lord? Initially,

I imagined that Mama was somewhere far, unreachable, and would be returning sometime soon.

The morning of her funeral finally came, and that morning I neglected to eat. In hindsight, that was the wrong move. I was tormented by the thought of burying my mother. It was the finality of it all that preoccupied my mind, and though I was pregnant, food was the farthest thing from my mind. As the celebration of life service came to an end, I walked behind her casket to the graveside.

As we walked towards the grave site for her burial, the reality finally came home to me that this was it and something began to expand in my chest. I knew what it was. It was the gaping hole that was there since I heard about Mama's death. It was getting ready to consume me. All efforts to contain it proved futile. The few objects I held (a cell phone, a program, and my nephew's jacket) were suddenly too heavy to bear. The pain then elevated to its crescendo and I surrendered to it. I let out another wail, this one was much louder, a much more visceral reflection of what was happening inside of me. It was different from the first wail because now Mama was actually gone, not hospitalized, and legitimized the need to scream.

There was so much power in letting it all out. It was freeing. Others rushed to my aid to make sure that in my episode of grief, I did not fall down causing injury to myself and my unborn child. The tears that flowed soothed the pain in my chest. It was a welcome release. Though my energy was spent, I am happy that I went through the long and torturous process of witnessing my mother's burial. This was the beginning of my healing.

My family's support went a very long way in my healing process. We were all struggling to cope with the loss. One of the ways we dealt with it was by coming together every chance we could get. My brother Damian moved back to Jamaica from Honduras, and my brother Karim came to my house every weekend. My sister Tricia and I were on the phone incessantly. She offered support and reassurance at every turn even during the times when she needed it. My Aunt Gae took some time off from work to come and help me to move into my new apartment in St. Ann as I created a nest to welcome my first-born child. She never left my side and she took care of me. The weight of the loss was outmatched by the level of support I received from my family and friends.

I never fully understood why God took Mama when He did, but I found things for which to be grateful.

On one of our many visits to the hospital, Mama passed out and I want to say she did in fact die. Remember how I told you earlier that my prayer life was completely propped up by her? As I stood by her bedside and looked at her with her face pale, her lips were a dark shade of purple and her hands were laying lifeless over her chest. This cannot be happening. Mama cannot die. All these thoughts came rushing in at the sight of her laying dead in front of me. I was desperate. That moment of desperation led to a gut-wrenching scream on the top of my lungs. It was a prayer and an SOS cry, "Jesus! Save Mi Madda!" After this outburst, the response was immediate. The color started coming back in Mama's face. Her lips came back to its normal colour and I noticed that Mama started to move. This was the very first day that I experienced for myself that God was real and that He answers prayers. In that moment, God was lifting my focus from my earthly mother to Himself.

When Mama died, my spiritual life was revitalized and the presence of God became a more amplified force in my life. The answered prayer was just one way in which I knew that God was going to be with me. The ministry of Auntie Gae, God's providential leading, and the feeling of not wanting to miss out on an opportunity to see my mother again are all great things that have emanated from the terrible ordeal of losing Mama.

Mama was scheduled to do a surgery the day after she passed. As my siblings stood around her bedside, she said, "I am going into surgery tomorrow; if I make it out alive, to God be the glory. And if I don't make it out alive, to God be the glory." When my brother shared these words with us, "To God be the Glory" became the theme of my life.

Memories of her selflessness, love for humanity, God-likeness, and integrity are being kept alive by my efforts to daily support my children on their own spiritual journeys so that they will one day claim the crown of life.

Having experienced the death of a mother, I have an increased sensitivity to what others who suffer similar losses are going through. Because of this, whenever I hear of a person losing their mom, I make a deliberate effort to minister to that individual with prayer and through words of encouragement.

I also share her story, a story of triumph over adversity and setbacks. It is a story of the transformative power of God's grace, a story of how a single mother gave her broken clay pot to the molder and shaper of her life. Then, in return, God gave her six biological children who are today living finding meaningful ways to advance the kingdom of God. I can't think of a more powerful way to expand her legacy than to allow her story to do the work of inspiring others to do the same.

Herein lies one of the answers on how we can re-shape and reframe the crises we face into a powerful source of empowerment and inspiration for others.

When the stories of our lives are being written, it is similar to a piece of painting. The most beautiful and captivating paintings are the ones possessing a variety of shades, tones, and textures pulled together as a powerful masterpiece. Whenever a painting is lacking one or all of these important elements, it runs the risk of looking unappealing and uninteresting.

The same is true with life. The peaks and valleys of our stories are all coming together in the hand of the master artist to create a grand masterpiece. If I was the artist of my own life, I may never have included the very dark shade of my mother's death. But what is the value of a work of art in my hand as opposed to the value of a piece of art in the hand of Michelangelo? Not much! God is our master artist. Your life's story is priceless in His hand, even the parts that are tough.

Our only duty as we are going through our crucible is to trust in His ability to produce a masterpiece. Like a blank canvas, place yourself at his disposal. We don't get to choose the parts of our stories that are only great to tell. All the experiences we endure and enjoy are meant to shape us into the masterpiece we can all become when our lives are being painted by the Master Artist where He is the one who gets to claim the glory for it all.

STEPS TOWARDS INTENTIONAL HEALING

Here are three things to help you navigate the loss of your mother:

1. Never repress your emotions. Whenever you feel the need to, cry. This has been proven to be a very helpful coping mechanism. There are some who will judge the manner in which you choose to do this, claiming that it is an inappropriate way to grieve someone who died in Christ. It is your unassailable right to shed tears and cry in order to relieve your own pain. No one has the right to tell you what volume or tone is appropriate to do so. If you continue to repress this, it will come out in other ways that are far more dangerous.

2. Embrace the support and outpouring of love that you receive from family and well-wishers. This is an essential part of our healing process. Sometimes, those who minister to us are also broken and you both need each other in order to heal. Sometimes, the way we choose to respond to others who are showing support during this time may help to facilitate their own healing in the process as well.

3. Share your story. Sharing your story changes your story. The more you talk about your story, the better you feel. Sharing also makes the loss much easier to bear. The benefits of doing this are manifold since others are also encouraged and inspired by your story.

RESOURCES

Instagram: https://www.instagram.com/apronsnheels

CHAPTER 15

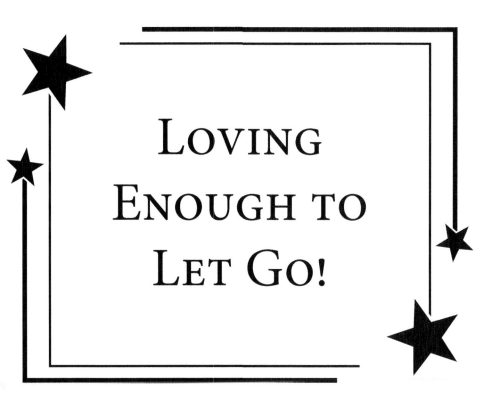

LOVING ENOUGH TO LET GO!

BY: JOY ALLEN

JOY ALLEN

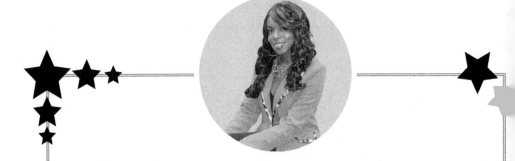

"To be absent from the body, is to be present with the Lord."
- 2 Corinthians 5:8

Yolanda "Joy" Allen, also known as The Joy Coach, is a four-time bestselling author (and counting), inspirational speaker, certified life & mental health coach, host, and emcee. Joy is also a certified speaker by Les Brown. She has studied Psychology and Christian Counseling at Liberty University and received several certifications as a life coach from Light University and the AACC American Association of Christian Counselors. As a certified Mental Health Coach and mental health advocate, her aim is to help others who struggle finding peace and joy in their lives due to lack of self-care and self-love, self-limiting beliefs, low self-esteem, self-doubt, depression, anxiety, abusive, toxic relationships, and more.

As an international inspirational speaker, Joy has spoken on various platforms, specifically on topics pertaining to mental health and wellness, self-care, self-love, domestic violence, and more. She has shared the stage with many phenomenal speakers, including her former coach and mentor, #1 motivational speaker Les Brown, as well as Dr. Forbes Riley.

Joy also runs a weekly room in her club on Clubhouse called the Joy Club and has her books as well as a new Inspirational line available on her website at TheJoyAllen.com.

Joy can also be reached for speaking engagements, hosting, and coaching services at TheJoycoach247@gmail.com

INTENTION

My intention is to show readers that we all go through some type of grief and can be affected by it in many ways; it is important to not try to go it alone or shut everyone out, but to allow God and others to give you the support and help you need to get through this process.

LOVING ENOUGH TO LET GO!

Being born in the sunshine state, I grew up in a pretty close-knit family. We had fun as kids; we actually went outside to play all day until the street lights came on, then we had to rush home before we got in trouble. Those were the good ole days! Kids these days would not know what to do if they went outside because they spend most of their days with their faces behind a screen. I remember my mom being such a talented woman and an amazing artist; she could fix anything, including cars. On top of that, she was an extremely beautiful woman.

It was the year 2002 and up until that point, I had been blessed to not have lost too many loved ones that were close to me with the exception of my grandmother. Well, all that was about to change. I had been living in Ohio for a while and decided to take a trip during spring break to go visit my family in Atlanta. Living in Atlanta was my dad's side of the family, my grandfather, my aunts, and cousins.

I had been there for a few days and really enjoyed being with the family; I was about to head back to Ohio when we got a call that my grandfather had been admitted to the hospital. So, we immediately all went to the VA Hospital where he was admitted. We all came together as a family. Some of my family flew into town and we were all there to be with him. One of the things I was grateful for was being able to spend some time alone with my grandfather; as I spent time with him, I prayed for him and he also prayed for himself as well.

Unfortunately, my grandfather died. It was really heartbreaking for us. He was the pillar of our family and now he is gone. So, our family went to Florida for my grandfather's funeral since that is where we are from. After my grandfather's funeral, I went to visit my mom and the rest of my family at my grandmother's house. It was good to see the rest of my family, although it was under unpleasant circumstances since the reason I was there in the first place was due to my grandfather's passing and funeral. I hadn't seen my mom in a few years, so I was glad to see her and the family. My mom had been having her own health challenges and I soon found out that she was not well. She had surgery on her legs months prior and was having severe pain and swelling, so something was definitely wrong with her.

We ended up taking my mom to the hospital, despite her reluctance; she did not want to go because she did not like hospitals. She and I have that in common due to a lot of the things that have transpired in the past. My aunt Mary and I were in the emergency room with my mom for hours before she was finally seen.

They were going to admit her, so we ended up leaving for the night. The next day, I went back to the hospital to check on my mom and for some reason instead of her being admitted for regular medical treatment, they had her in the psychiatric unit. I was livid! I went and spoke to her doctor after seeing my mom. I asked her why was my mom not admitted for medical treatment as that is why we brought her there in the first place? The doctor said that my mom was not actually physically sick and she was just exaggerating! "Are you serious?" I asked. I responded to her that the reason we brought her here was for a physical condition and that my mom was sick! I then told her, I had seen her swollen legs and feet that were causing her pain, so does that mean I am exaggerating too?

After a few days, I ended up returning to Ohio and I was appointed my mother's Power Of Attorney (POA). Not even a week later, I got a call and guess who it was? It was the same doctor I spoke to that admitted my mom to the psychiatric unit. She said, "Oh I am calling to let you know that you were right, your mom was really sick! I am sorry. We had to admit her to the medical unit." Those words have haunted me for years. It was not that the doctors cannot help people; it is just that some of them choose not to help for whatever reasons they conjure. I truly feel that this doctor came to her own conclusions and did not care to listen to my mom or myself and hear our concerns.

Things went from bad to worse. I continued getting calls from the hospital weekly. Every week, there was another issue. She ended up getting pneumonia, then gangrene was setting in and they had to do an amputation on her leg to prevent it from spreading through the rest of her body. Although they mentioned the surgery to me, they failed to communicate the same information to my mother. After the surgery, she woke up thinking it was a simple procedure only to discover it was not. After her surgery, they had her transferred to a nursing home for rehabilitation due to the amputation and unfortunately that was a nightmare in itself. Her experience there was not the greatest, as she was neglected and mistreated and did not receive the best of care. My Aunt Mary acted as my eyes and ears and would keep me abreast of the situation with my mom; she would visit her regularly to check on her and update me. One day, I got a disturbing call from my aunt about my mom, and she told me that my mom was outside in her wheelchair, left unattended, and she was attacked by wasps. She was stung repeatedly and yelled for help and no one came to help her for a while. My aunt said that when she went to see her, my mom was completely shut down and told her that when she was put back in her bed, there were still wasps in her clothes. To make matters worse, we eventually found out that due to the neglect at the nursing home and lack of care, my mom had developed bedsores the size of grapefruits! This was due to them not properly turning her or cleaning her as they should. Her condition led to her being hospitalized again.

With everything that was happening, I knew I needed to spend time with my mom as the reports were not good. Her health declined rapidly. I got on a plane with my then 2 year old daughter and headed back to Florida to care for my mom. After my mom's treatment in the hospital, they had done all they could do and transferred her to another nursing facility for care. By this time, her condition had gotten progressively worse and she was not doing well. The next several weeks were some of the most difficult times of my life and hers as I helped to care for her. I prayed and I was confident that she was going to be healed.

There are many stages of grief, and not everyone experiences them all the same. I know for me, one of the major stages I recall was denial. I was in denial about my mom dying for a while. I was believing God to heal her for a while and not accepting the fact that she could possibly die. I guess that's where faith came in and I was not sure if it was all faith or some of that was the fact that I was unwilling to accept my mom may actually not be here anymore. It was a gospel song that actually helped me to finally accept the fact that my mom was dying.

Grief is a natural and healthy response to loss. During the grieving process, we may experience all kinds of difficult and uncomfortable emotions, from shock and confusion to anxiety and depression. Though working through grief can be messy and complicated, it most often resolved naturally over time and is a necessary part of processing, and ultimately accepting, the loss that we have experienced.

There are 5 stages of grief: denial, anger, bargaining, depression, and acceptance. Everyone's experience may not be the same and they may not experience it in that particular order. With the experience with my mom, I experienced denial first, as I was basically in denial with the fact that my mom was dying. Then, I experienced bargaining where I prayed to God and asked him to heal my mom and in return I would testify about how He practically brought her back from the brink of death and healed her.

The next stage I experienced was acceptance and here is the story of how that occurred. My mom had been growing weaker and weaker and her body was basically deteriorated from the gangrene; at this point, she was halfway gone. I still hadn't completely accepted the fact that she was dying and wouldn't be here any longer.

That Sunday, I went to my Aunt Mary's church. Someone sang a song by Yolanda Adams called "In The Midst of it All." The words to that song really ministered to my soul and all of the emotion and reality of my mom's condition set in. All of the emotion I had been holding back poured out as I burst into tears as God literally spoke to me through that song. He told me it was going to be okay, that my mom would be taken care of, and that I had nothing to worry about. It was at that moment that a sudden peace came over me and that was the moment I finally "accepted" my mom's death.

After watching her dealing with the pain and suffering she had been going through for months and spending six weeks caring for her, it became my pain as well. But as the song said, "God kept me." It was not an easy task, but I felt like God literally put a shield over me to protect my mind, heart, and emotions as I cared for my mom, especially with the condition her body was in. This was not an easy task, as some of the nursing staff couldn't even bear seeing her condition. I know it was nothing but God who gave me the strength and the ability to do it, especially for such a long period of time.

So, after church, I went to the nursing home to see my mom. I told her it was okay to "let go." The next morning, I woke up and went into prayer and asked God if it would be too much for me to handle mentally, to take my mom before I got there – as I knew she was dying soon. When I got up and walked to the door, my grandmother told me she was gone. The Lord allowed me to experience good grief and lessened the pain by not putting more on me than I could bear; He took my mother out of her pain and suffering.

One thing I know is that a lot of times, our loved ones will try to "hold on" for us. Despite how much it may hurt to "stay" and how they may want to let go and move on, they know that doing so may be a lot for us and they may fight to stay for our sake. I believe that when we "release" them, it gives them the sense of peace they need to stop fighting to stay here and move on to the next phase in life which as a believer, I believe is in Heaven with Jesus Christ.

Having a strong support system is so crucial when dealing with grief. One of the things I did personally was seek God, pray, and meditate. Going to church and getting support from family and friends is also helpful. Joining a support group is a great option as well, as you will find other people in the same or similar situation you can talk to.

Steps Towards Intentional Healing

There are many things you can do to help with grief. First of all, know you are not alone. There are many people who have or are experiencing the same thing you are, so don't hesitate to reach out for help when needed. Other helpful tips are as follows:

- Acknowledge your pain and accept the fact that grief can trigger many different and unexpected emotions.

- Understand that your grieving process will be unique to you; don't expect it to be the same as someone else's. Do not compare your healing, processing journey, and timeline to someone else's. Allow yourself the time you need to grieve and heal.

- Take care of yourself and get the support from loved ones, and seek therapy if needed. Seek out face-to-face support from people who care about you.

Resources

Instagram: @ JOYCOACH247

LinkTree : TheJoyCoach

Website: TheJoyAllen.com

CHAPTER 16

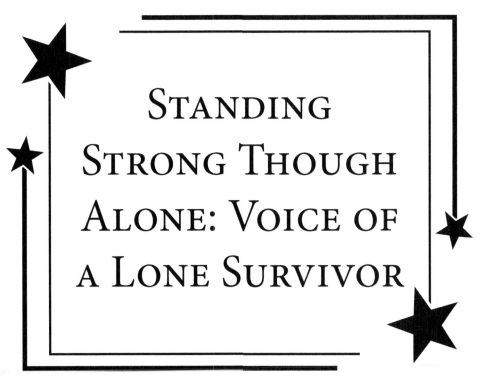

STANDING STRONG THOUGH ALONE: VOICE OF A LONE SURVIVOR

By: **DR. PAULENE GAYLE-BETTEN**

DR. PAULENE GAYLE-BETTEN

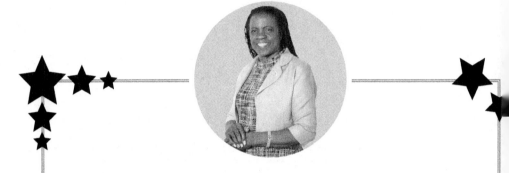

Rejoicing in hope; patient in tribulation, continuing in prayer.
- Romans 12:12
"Today's encouragement and advice become tomorrow's strength." -
Paulene Gayle-Betten (2022)

Dr. Paulene Gayle-Betten, hails from the parish of St. Catherine, Jamaica. Being brought up in a farming community shaped her experience and helped her navigate the early struggles associated with living in a farming community and educational achievement.

Dr. Gayle-Betten is an Educator, Sociologist, Trainer, and Researcher. She is a graduate of the University of the West Indies with an earned Bachelor of Arts degree in History, a Master's degree in Sociology, and a PhD in Education and Leadership from Northern Caribbean University where she served as an Assistant Professor prior to accepting the challenge as principal of Hagley Park Prep School where she has been serving since August 30, 2016. Dr. Gayle-Betten is actively involved in community work and currently provides volunteer service with the Jamaica Red Cross as a member of the Psychosocial Support (PSS) Team. She also serves as Public Relations Officer (PRO) for the Citizens Association in her Community.

INTENTION

I hope as you read my story you will realize that it takes courage to navigate grief. This experience of death and loss can help you as it has helped me to discover emotional power and strength that I never thought I had. Whenever you are faced with demanding situations, such as illness, you pray for healing but do not always get the results you crave. Therefore, embracing the reality of the worst-case scenario will give you the strength to stand even when the results are unfavorable.

STANDING STRONG THOUGH ALONE: VOICE OF A LONE SURVIVOR

I was lucky my sister, Beck, and I were close; we shared a bond second to none. There were five of us as children, but my older brothers and sister had moved away from home so Beck and I had the time of our lives. The childhood memories are indelibly etched in my mind and held in the formation of thoughts that would have shaped my experience.

As time progressed, Beck moved away from home, first to Kingston and eventually to the United States of America. Years later, I acquired a visa so I could visit her. Together we shared long summer holidays, weekends, and vacations, sharing the same bed and more; those were treasured moments. Beck was the life of the party; she walked into a room and it immediately lit up. Her beam of fragrance engulfs the atmosphere. She was the bedrock of the family, kind, caring, and having the welfare of everyone at heart.

My drive to continue my education and to make a better and more meaningful contribution to society was fuelled by her support and encouragement. This influenced me to seek educational opportunities. My journey through Teachers' colleges and Universities rewarded me with a Diploma, a Masters, and eventually a PhD. I often look back at my life and try to measure my achievements. I understand now that God had a plan for my life, but I just did not know how it would unfold. On one of my many travels to the United States to visit my sister, I brought her a book entitled A Sister is a Very Special Friend. The book is an anthology of poems edited by Robin Andrews. The title of the book described Beck well because she was indeed "my special friend."

Kristy Jorgensen did a great description of Beck in her poem, even though the two never crossed paths. "You are the most Beautiful Person I know – not just outside but inside too, you have a wonderful sense of humor, a loyalty that not many people have, and the gift of love you give to others." Thank you, Kristy; that is my sister, Beck.

Words really cannot explain, and the space allotted here is insufficient to capture the fantastic wonders and fragrance of a special sister and the friendship we shared. Life was certainly great!

As Elbert Hubbard said, "When life gives you lemons, make lemonade." The year 2019 will remain indelibly etched in my book of memories. I had more than enough lemons to make lemonade for the entire family. It was a devastating moment as I watched Beck take her last breath. The gift of life was no more for her, and I said a tearful goodbye. With teary eyes, I realized that it was no ordinary goodbye; I now must live without her. Suddenly I was hit by a gigantic lemon that insistently engulfed my thoughts and I pondered. I am now physically alone, but was I?

I vividly recall a niece who had passed, and on the day of the preparation for her burial, her son died. That was a blow below the belt, the loss of two family members a few days apart. Then later on, life threw another huge lemon. Mickel, another nephew who was only 26 years old, came to Jamaica for his wedding in March of 2016, and in less than two weeks after returning to the United States, he died. Recount with me. My first encounter with death came at about age 9 when I lost my mother. The death of my dad was upsetting too, but then I had my brothers' and sisters' shoulders on which to lean. I was close to my dad, so I missed him dearly. Fast forward to the year 2015, which was the beginning of a series of losses and sorrow that significantly impacted my life.

Imagine losing all your siblings in quick succession. I call it the number game. There were five. On February 14, 2015, my favorite brother left us after a few days of illness. Then there were four. I felt as though my heart was ripped apart and I was knocked down once more. I was barely coming to terms with the loss of this brother and then had to deal with the death of another brother and a sister, on May 23 and December 13, 2017, respectively. Then there were two, two girls to tell the tales. My sister relocated to Florida, and we envisioned doing many things together, such as shopping sprees, cruises, lunch, and dinner dates. The date August 6, 2019 came like a roaring, starving lion. Short-lived was my dream of bonding and having a good life with my sister. As I watched her take her last breath, I had to swallow the frog. Now there was one. Everything ended prematurely; indeed I was knocked down.

Having lost my mother at such a tender age and stage of development, I was bolstered with capabilities to stand alone, yet not alone for there were many, including dad and my siblings. I never fully understood what happened; all I knew was that my mother was no longer home, and a piece of the puzzle was missing. The frequent occurrences of death in my family were unfathomable and overwhelming. Death was a norm in my family, to the extent that whenever I shared about the death of a family member with anyone, their immediate response would be, "Again!"

My socio-emotional faculties underwent much pressure because I was intricately involved in the organizing of funerals and reading eulogies or remembrances. At one of the many funerals, one of my nieces said, "Auntie, when I die, I want you to read my eulogy." At that moment, I thought my emotions were being attacked and I immediately reprimanded her for making such an utterance.

However, my experience with death/loss would have molded, shaped, and prepared my feelings to deal with the loss of family members, one after the other. In 2015, I lost my brother. The year 2017 brought a double dose of death taking two of my siblings, one at the beginning and the other at the end of the year. I was torn, yet I found the strength to take the lead in making funeral arrangements. This was no easy task, but I realized that other members of the family needed the kind of support that I had to offer. This was also my soul-searching moment as I asked for God's leading and directives for the remainder of the journey. In 2019, two years later, the carpet was swept from under my feet, leaving 'A lone survivor.'

My life has been a journey, and I navigated with many hurts, tears, and a sorrowful heart. Along the way, I learned several positive lessons. Mixed emotions still linger, but instead of re-living the hurt and pain associated with death, I stand alone empowered today to retell my story. My early encounter with death certainly prepared me to face the difficulties of future loss.

My first task, after the loss of my sister Beck, was that of acceptance. I accepted the fact that my sister was no longer with me and that I was the lone survivor of the siblings. For sure, it was difficult at first, but I asked God to give me the courage to accept the things I cannot change. Once I got to the place where I understood my reality, I had to face it and the baggage that it brought.

Positive self-talk was my next step. I questioned myself, I talked aloud, and then made a list of the things I needed to do. I even asked myself, what if the shoe were on the other foot, what would my sister do? I know for sure that she would do all she could to ensure that everything is done decently and orderly. My self-talk includes all the things I know would make her happy and take pleasure in getting them done. During the process, I gave myself several self-directives. Through the loss of my sister, I learned the art of self-talk, which works well, particularly in situations such as those that unfolded in my story.

Shared experience was another element that I found to be useful in helping to bring healing and comfort. I found sharing to be therapeutic. The more I talk with others about the situation, the less difficult it becomes. Moreover, I enjoy sharing the memories of a wonderful sister and it sure makes me feel empowered.

Grief is not easily shared or expected but earlier in my journey, I was privileged to encounter the work of Dr. Grace A. Kelly in her book Grieve If You Must: A 21-day Plan for Grieving Healing and Restoration, in which she shared her grieving experience and outlined ways in which others can overcome theirs. I remember contributing to the title not realizing that it would have been a significant source of strength in navigating my grief.

Can you recall when Joseph's brothers were angry with him because of his dreams? Yet, when they came face to face with Joseph in Egypt, they thought that he would be angry with them; instead, Joseph reassured them, "As for you, you meant evil against me, but God meant it for good in order to bring about this present result, to preserve many people alive" (Genesis 50:20).

Such was my situation, being angry at God for taking my siblings, especially Beck; I could not see the good for which I was being preserved. Today I am more empathetic towards others.

My journey through death and loss has helped me to use my experience to encourage others and help them to face the reality of life's lemons that are likely to come at them. Through it all, I am grateful that I am still alive and that I did not pass on before my sister, Beck. When I saw her suffering, I found the courage to face God. I prayed, "God I don't want to die and leave my sister in this condition." By now, you would have realized that is an answered prayer. Today I am no longer angry with God, for I am now appreciative of my crucibles that have contributed to my resilience.

I reminisce on my tragic experiences with the death and loss of my siblings and wish they were here, but that is something I cannot change. At Beck's funeral, I cried, "I want my sister back." Repeatedly, I cried those words. My understanding of death would have taught me that Beck could not come back, so why was I repeating those words? It was there, in a quiet moment away from everyone, that I asked God to grant me the courage to accept the things I cannot change, which He did.

The dramaturgical events leading to the loss of two brothers and two sisters within four years, have molded me to embrace the strength enfolded in my reality. Often friends and family members would ask, "How is it that you are able to talk so freely about your situation?" I learned strength of character, and it was demonstrated in my being empathetic and caring towards persons who are experiencing or would have experienced similar situations.

Being bold in the face of adversities has shaped my character and helped me to face challenging situations, inclusive of death. Strength is laced with courage, but fear can cripple your strength. Therefore, my situation helped me to release fear and grasp the hand of strength, a principle I have been using in all areas of life.

I was empowered when someone with whom I recently shared my experience told me that the encouragement and advice I had shared with her had helped her in a remarkable way to face the reality of the loss of her husband. That is something I want to do: use the memories of those I love to empower others so that they, too, can navigate through their pain and loss.

The use of this medium to share my story points me to another source of empowerment, that of writing. Writing provides the opportunity to explore and share my story in a more organized manner without reliving the hurt. The story never ends though, since empowerment is not a short-term phenomenon; it is part of what you do on a daily basis. When you are empowered by what you do for others, your positive energy increases and exposes the good feeling.

I utilize my experiences from the traumatic situations to take control of my own life. I understand that empowerment requires action rather than intention, and as such, I transformed my intention into action by serving others.

The feeling one experiences as a result of death and loss cannot be explained in any descriptive manner even though the situation might be similar; everyone will share a unique experience. When faced with adversities, pull from your spiritual reservoir. Remember, you might be alone in your physical space but never doubt for a second that someone else is present in your space. Take time out to do some self -talks. Walk around by yourself and assess the situation. Now that you have done that, ask yourself which piece of the puzzle is missing? In other words, find yourself. What is your worth in this situation? What action do you need to take? Sometimes you must take the lemons that life offers and make your own lemonade. As you face your loss, remember Ephesians 6:10, which states, "Be strong in the Lord and in the power of His might."

Steps Towards Intentional Healing

As the saying by Clayton M. goes, "There is no one-size-fits-all approach that anyone can offer." However, as you heal intentionally and navigate your scars, here are three things that have helped me traverse my dark valleys. These might help you to do the same.

Acceptance. Accept the fact that the person(s) you lost is/are no longer with you. For sure, it will be difficult at first, but pray and ask God to give you the courage to accept the things you cannot change. Once you get to the place where you understand that reality, you will be ready for your healing and new normal.

Positive Self-Talk. This has been proven to make one feel good about themselves and has served to encourage and motivate people to keep going amidst the odds. This also helps to reduce symptoms of depression, anxiety, risk of self-harm and suicide, improves self-esteem, and aid with stress management.

Shared Experience. This is also useful in helping to bring healing and comfort in a caring community. It is therapeutic. The more you talk with others about the situation, the less difficult it becomes for you to manage and you do not have to do it alone. In your sharing, focus on sharing memories that preserve the legacy of lives well lived.

Resources

Linkedin: Paulene Gayle Betten

Liketree: https://linktr.ee pgaylebetten

CHAPTER 17

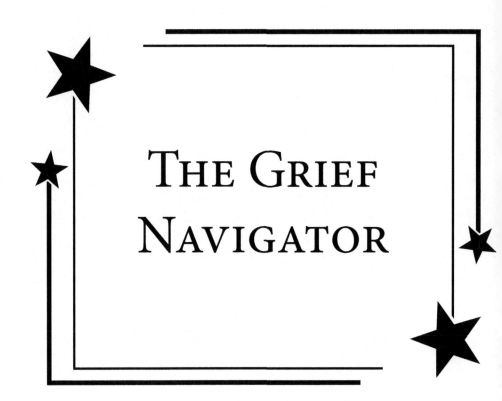

THE GRIEF NAVIGATOR

By: **Dr. Grace A. Kelly**

Dr. Grace A. Kelly

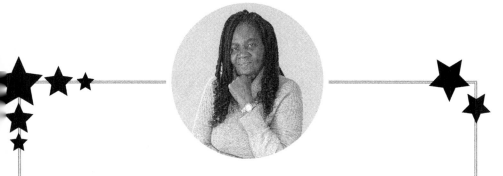

"Grieving is to pain as breathing is to life, so Grieve if you must."
- Dr. Grace Kelly (2010)

Dr. Grace A. Kelly counselor, educator, international motivational speaker, Restorative Justice Practitioner, and Crisis Interventionist is also a five-time Amazon best-selling author, Her experience of navigating her way through her own grief, as well as her academic preparation, qualifies her to be an effective world-renown grief and bereavement, therapist coach.

With over 30 years of progressive support to individuals, families, and community members, in governmental and non-governmental community-based organizations, schools and churches across the islands of the Caribbean, North America, and Europe, she has learned to be tolerant of personal and cultural differences. Being the 2019 Governor-General Achievement Awardee for the parish of Manchester, validated the value of her work in nation-building. Testament to her passion and purpose is her book titled Grieve If You Must: A 21-day Plan for Grieving, Healing, and Restoration. She is the host of Let's Talk Life and Legacy: A Moment with Dr. Grace aired on her YouTube Channel – Facing Life and Facebook. She also hosts the Healing Stars: From Scars to Stars Podcast. Her mission is to operate a comprehensive support system for individuals, and families to grieve intentionally, heal deliberately, navigate their grief and learn how to achieve and maintain a worthwhile life.

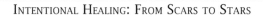

INTENTION

Everyone, intentionally and unintentionally, is scarred at some point in their life. You may not cause it but you can not escape it. Scars come from many sources. Grief, being a common source, is a natural phenomenon that transcends age, gender, nationality, race, creed, educational status, religious affiliation or convictions. Grief is real, inescapable, and sure. As certain as there is life, there is pain, and our natural reaction to pain is grief. Grief does not need permission to happen but as you journey with me you will find that there is always a way to successfully navigate grief. Cheer up and be of good courage. My story, Grief Navigator, is designed to give you a reason to hope that there is life after grief.

THE GRIEF NAVIGATOR

Growing up in a family of ten--four boys, four girls, and our parents--was an adventure. I am not saying we never had challenges, but we surmounted any challenges and obstacles with a praying mother of faith. We struggled, yet with Mama being around, we had a good life despite the dynamic mysteries of an absentee father. Recounting some of the most amazing aspects of our life in the early days always brings a sense of laughter and joy. Mama was small in stature but a giant of a woman. She was so powerful, she commanded the respect of everyone. The moral compass was not only applied when we were at home but was equally applicable at work and in the community. That meant we could not go anywhere or do anything without a report coming back to her. I recall wanting to be "bad" but was saved by the thought of Mama finding out. Family worship was mandatory and if we chose not to get up, our sleep was interrupted by the melodious voice singing as if a whole congregation was present. Scouting through the field for the seasonal fruits was more exciting than attending to my daily chores, but you know who paid if the latter was not done.

August 1983, was my 09-11. That Wednesday morning, I stood by the bed in tears, and lamentation over our obvious lack. My discerning mother saw and felt my pain. Mama and I were so connected that, at times, I was convinced that she was hearing my thoughts and would always respond accurately. She turned toward me and said, "Don't worry, God is going to help me to help all of you." And without a moment's pause, she, with her gaze fixed towards heaven, said, "If you come back on Sunday and don't see me, don't cry. I'm gone home." I instantly felt my life source dry up. I held mama in my embrace. Please, Mama, you can't leave me; you are my life, my conscience, my breath. How could I live without you?

A few moments passed, and I was still beside the bed and Mama at the back door. With a rapidly palpitating heart, breathlessness, hands soaked with perspiration, and trembling knees, I turned and said, "See you Sunday, Mama." Evidently, I was denying the inevitable, as I left for Mandeville, Manchester, to attend the Festival of the Laity, a celebratory function of the Inter-American Division of Seventh-day Adventists. Mama remained true to her word in life and at death.

On doctor's orders, we were en route to Cornwall Regional Hospital, Montego Bay St. James, Jamaica. Mama mustered every ounce of breath and said, "Gre." Excited, I leaned over and placed my ear close to her mouth. She continued, "Greee, Greeee, Greeeeeeeeeeee," her last attempt to call my name faded with a penetrating release of her last warm moist breath that, caressed my ears, and disturbed my emotions. Returning that Sunday, finding Mama unresponsive and almost unrecognizable, just a semblance of her in the bed, rested with me for a long time. I gently closed her eyes to block her glaring, penetrating stare, which spoke volumes to me.

We were literally traveling on a rough and winding road falling into potholes. That was no match to the upsurge of emotions. A hurricane like the September 1988 Gilbert, which was identified as the most destructive storm in the history of Jamaica, was an easy breeze compared to the tumultuous uproar of my emotions. My heart sank through to my feet and all my internal organs were knitted together like a ball of yarn. Upon arriving at the hospital emergency entrance, my knees wobbled as I exited the ambulance. I cried so loudly that heaven heard and responded but there was not a sound coming from my mouth. The earth stood still yet it felt as if I was caught in a whirlwind. God, what is this that Thou hath done unto me?

The moment Mama died, my life left me. I was knocked down and out on the battlefield of life. Needless to say, I went into overdrive. I was speechless and motionless. I was convinced that life could not continue without my mama. I was angry with God, myself, and worst of all, my father. I resented anyone and anything that would remind me of my loss. Overwork and busyness became my opium. I shunned every opportunity to be in the presence of any trigger. I was left with pain, agony, confusion, and the desire not to live.

The emotional pain inflicted on me by this loss was unquestionably the most traumatic and horrendous I have ever experienced. This chapter is far too limited to narrate how I navigated such a scar that caused me to grieve for what seemed like a lifetime, punctuated with stints of hopelessness, anger, depression, and despair. When Mama died, my passion for life ended. On the day of her funeral, I was told that it took six strong men to remove me from her sepulchre to make way for her body to be laid to rest.

How I navigated this scar is still a mystery to me. In 2007, after a series of deaths, including my sister Olive on October 1. I knew I had to do something. I was at that time teaching Techniques of Counselling at both the graduate and undergraduate levels. The undergraduate text was Intentional Interviewing and Counseling by Allen E, Ivey and Mary Bradford Ivey. Fascinated by the concept of intentionality which I found very useful in my class activities and counseling practice when I was in the darkest hours of my grief and did not know if there was a way out, I decided to try a new thing--be intentional about healing my scars. I assigned myself as my client, as I would pair the students in my class to treat one another's presenting problems.

Their presenting problems could have been made-up but mine was real. Using my concentric grief circle in the Day Two Activity of my book, I listed the six most painful things that caused much grief. Then I ranked them in order, based on the level of intensity–very low to extremely high–moving from the outer to the inner circle. The final pain point identified as the sixth and the highest level of intense pain was the death of my sister Olive. That sunk through all other pain points to the core of the most severe, which, of course, was my mother's death. Olive's death caused a volcanic interruption of emotions. My life was a mess. I felt like running, but my feet were fixed to the ground, and my head, like a whirlwind, spun out of control. Somehow, I knew then that I had to face everything and rise.

My scars covered me like a well-done, full-body tattoo. How did I navigate such scars? I scheduled times to grieve. During that time, I embraced my loss and memorialized my mother. I designed a 21-day treatment plan for me, applying a three-stage formula for grieving, healing, and restoration. Using that formula, accompanied by the skills, techniques, and the recommended guide by Ivey & Ivey, and practising micro shifts and positive habit stocking I got better at managing my grief. That process became my guide and led me toward a healthier and more fulfilling way of life.

I later realized that resilience, developed from all the pain and grief I suffered, is interwoven into the fiber of who I have become. I am the product of my past, which informs my calling, passion, and purpose. One of my original quotes in 2010 says it best: "Grieving is to pain as breathing is to life. If you want to live you breathe, if you want to heal you grieve, so grieve if you must." The early mention that life could not go on without my mother and that my world would not be a safe space would be classified as catastrophizing. I was always thinking the worst would happen. Today, instead of magnifying the memories as triggers for pain and grief, I now accept them as reminders to memorialize Mama's legacy.

I am now at the point of celebrating her life instead of mourning her death. I recognize that "grief is the price we pay for love" and the degree to which I loved her was equal to the degree I am grieving her death. I am most grateful and value my mother for being given a second chance at life in the early 1960 so that I could have been born, after her miraculous "resurrection". For this I am grateful. My whys have now been translated into praise and adoration to God for His mercies and for Mama's lasting legacy of integrity, self-respect, and other respect, charity, compassion, prayer, and thanksgiving.

One statement from my professional bio, aptly represents who I have become as a direct result of my having navigated so many scars. It says: "As a counselor and educator, Dr. Kelly's life has influenced the lives of many as she seeks to empower every person with whom she interacts in becoming self-fulfilled. She is a role model for both young and old and has been a strong source of support to many who applaud her for her humility, sincerity, and her understanding heart".

I'm not sure what you hear or see when you read this, but I sense empathy, courage, and dedication are but a few character development elements. As a result of the impact of my scars, I have vowed that as long as I can help in any way, no one should have to suffer such pain as I have. My work as a grief and bereavement therapist/coach is birthed out of my scars. I now accept triggers, which I once avoided as formulae for developing treatment plans and programmes to support grieving individuals and their families.

This particular story is about navigating grief scars throughout my lifetime. I have been riddled with pain from the many grief situations by which I was knocked down flat–countless times. This is why I write, publish, speak, and support individuals, families, and communities to navigate scars as they seek to heal intentionally. Thousands of persons have already benefitted from my direct intervention and training in grief management. The recent establishment of The Olive Branch Global LLC, is my way of honoring my mother and my sister Olive's legacy as I lead a body of subject-matter experts in providing training, consultation, coaching, writing, and other services designed to empower persons to be actualized and self-fulfilled. This is a safe space where grieving persons find hope, and lasting peace; where pain is translated into passion, purpose, and profit.

If you have read to this point, it means you sense that there is hope. With God at your side and this book of stories in your hand, never again will you have to walk your journey alone. Grief is sometimes presented to us as a giant, untamable monster, an interference rather than an intrinsic part of life. But I assure you that if I navigated my scars and worked through my grief, you can also.

I leave you with these thoughts expressed by Queen Elisabeth II. "Grief is the price we pay for love." So your grief will most likely be at the same level of intensity as your love. Psalm 34:18 says, "The Lord is near to the brokenhearted and saves the crushed in spirit." Trust Him to save you. You can also release your burdens to Him. He has the capacity to handle all of your cares if you only let Him. And finally, "Grieving is to pain as breathing is to life, so grieve if you must."

INTENTIONAL HEALING: FROM SCARS TO STARS

Steps Towards Intentional Healing

Here is a three-phase approach designed to be used by grieving persons to navigate to the hope side of their grief: Grieve deliberately, heal intentionally, and be restored.

Grieve Intentionally: Grieving is a natural reaction to pain. Grieving is the process of how we react to our perception of any loss. This is the most feared among all steps, toward intentional grieving, yet most essential. Most persons usually seek to manage pain. But managing pain may not be grieving. In fact, contrary to popular belief, it is the tendency to view grieving only as an emotional experience, with only symptoms of emotional pain and distress, but this is faulty because grief does have a physical component. Grief also threatens our physical health. Because those physical symptoms can be treated with injections and other medications, one can effectively manage pain without grieving but will not experience holistic healing. Being intentional about treating your scars can allow you to grieve until it becomes as seamless as breathing.

Heal Deliberately: Healing speaks to the process of becoming healthy after experiencing pain. Being deliberate is defined as being done consciously and intentionally, being careful and unhurried, and engaging in long and careful consideration. An easy and accurate conclusion is that healing is not an overnight rushed process. Take time and schedule grieving time.

Be Open To True Restoration: Restoration is the act of returning to a former state or condition that is the hallmark of this process needed to heal intentionally. It does not need a qualifier and is absolutely necessary for one to experience and live a healthy, fulfilled life amidst grief. Is it easy? No! Absolutely not! Is it worth it? Most certainly.

Resources

Linktree: https://linktr.ee/drgraceak

Website: www.theolivebranchglobal.llc

YouTube: https://www.youtube.com/c/FacingLife

CHAPTER 18

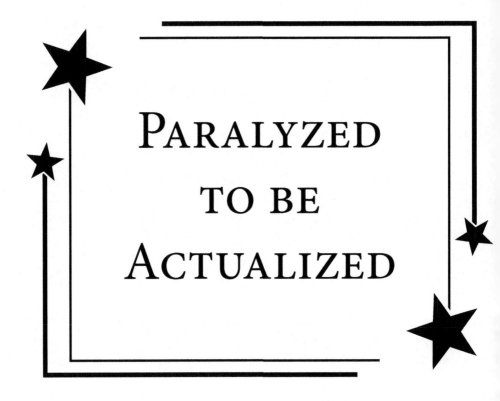

PARALYZED
TO BE
ACTUALIZED

BY: DR. IVANAH THOMAS

Dr. Ivanah Thomas

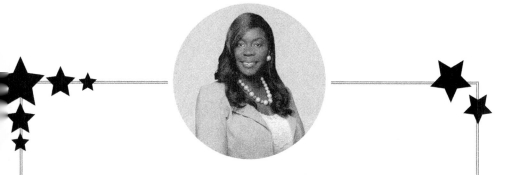

"Let no one break you; they did not make you. You are God's masterpiece." - I. Thomas, 2022

Dr. Ivanah Thomas is a Medical Doctor in addition to holding three other Doctoral degrees in Clinical Psychology, Philosophy, and Theology. She also holds a Master's in Business Administration-MBA, and a current Registered Nurse License in the state of Florida. Her long illustrious career in the healthcare industry spans over three decades. She has an unquenchable desire for service to humanity, seeking to especially serve the disenfranchised, hurting, and sick across the globe. Her passion for service has led her to serve in many countries including Ghana, Nigeria, Guatemala, Costa Rica, and other Caribbean countries.

She's a dynamic motivational speaker. In 2019 she was invited twice by the United Nations in New York to speak on issues affecting girls and women globally and on unique ways of empowering rural families.

She's a committed God's Girl and remains a dedicated humanitarian, with a zeal to empower others to excavate their authentic selves and relentlessly pursue their Divine destinies.

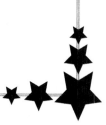

INTENTION

My purpose for sharing my story is to first give glory to God for His unquestionable faithfulness and to give hope to you who have experienced debilitating, life-altering circumstances, the nature of which threatens the very fibers of your existence and destiny. It is my hope that when you hear or read my story, you would realize that there is purpose in your pain and that no matter how awful the circumstances you have endured or are still going through, God specializes in turning horrible situations into platforms of greatness for His glory. My story commenced with the hallmarks and underpinnings of great pain on every level, but through God's divine providence, it has culminated into an unimaginably rich tapestry of grace and beauty.

PARALYZED TO BE ACTUALIZED

It was a beautiful Thursday afternoon in June with the hot Jamaican sun beaming through the majestic mango tree that sits at the front of our little wooden house. It was the summer holidays after completing grade six in elementary school. Summer was just the greatest time of the year for me, as that was when I would get to go spend the holidays with my grandparents in Manchester, fondly called 'country.' As I played the game hopscotch with my four siblings, I heard the all too familiar voice of my dad bellowing out mine and my mom's name to come quickly. I had never heard such excitement in my dad's voice. I hurriedly dashed off to meet him in front of our home, but Mom had made it to him before I did.

As I emerged at the front of the house, my eyes caught the most amazing and proud look I had ever seen on my dad's face as he stood with the newspaper in his hand. I was wondering what was the excitement all about but before I could ask what happened, my dad shouted, "You pass your exam and you are going to Glenmuir High School." My adorable mom, not to be outdone, said, "Henry, let me see the paper." I watched in utter amazement as he pointed out my name to her and said, "See it there, she pass, my daughter pass for Glenmuir. Bev, I told you she would pass."

My mom instantly let out the loudest squeals of sheer joy I have ever heard from her, that even the neighbors came running over. This meant that I had gained a placement in one of the most prestigious high schools in Jamaica. The rest of the day was just some of the happiest moments in my childhood as I watched my parents beam with such joy and pride at my accomplishment. For the first time, I was given the privilege of getting one bottle of Cola Champagne soda and a whole beef patty with a coco bread for myself. Growing up with four siblings meant back then that we shared almost everything, including food, but not that day; it was my day and my parents' way of celebrating me. Oh, the happiness of that day still brings a big smile to my face.

The exhilarating journey of being in high school with a doting, supportive dad was abruptly interrupted in a way that would change the trajectory of my life forever. It was mid-October 1983, in my Junior-4th year of high school when one day I received the dreadful news that my beloved dad had suddenly passed away at home. I remember rushing home with my heart pounding faster than the swift feet of a cheetah to see my dad. I arrived home to find his lifeless body stretched out on the floor in his bedroom. I immediately collapsed to the floor clutching his cold, lifeless body as tears like a torrential downpour flowed from my eyes. The horror of grief gripped my tremulous body as a flood of thoughts and emotions raced uncontrollably through my mind. My mom was now living overseas and I was the oldest of five siblings; oh how life was about to change. I quickly realized that all the dreams my dad had for me and how he would proudly represent me at my graduation were now dashed forever.

I stumbled through the next two and a half months, grappling with the immense loss of my hero, my biggest cheerleader, and defender, my amazing dad. It was Christmas Eve 1983, but the festivity of the season could not begin to fill the enormity of the gaping hole in my heart left by Dad's sudden passing. Life indeed was rapidly changing, and as horrible as things had been since the passing of my dad, it was about to disintegrate into an unimaginable abyss of pain and darkness. On Christmas Eve, just two and a half months after my dad's sudden passing, whilst I was still in the throes of grief, I was raped at knife point. The appalling, terrifying experience left me in a state of shock, anger, and a multiplicity of emotions as my person and my life were ravaged by a savage. To add insult to injury, the horrifying experience compounded my pain, as not only was I violated in the worst way, but I was now pregnant from the assault. The physician strongly encouraged my mom to allow me to terminate the pregnancy, but it was a decision my mom couldn't make despite the circumstances. Therefore, I had no choice; I had to drop out of high school and prepare to become a teen mom.

When my dad passed away suddenly, I felt a part of me died that day; but then after being assaulted and faced with the new reality of carrying a child, being a child myself, threw me into a pit of sorrow, shock, anger, shame, and depression that I thought for sure there was no way out. I cried myself to sleep every night, and daily the thoughts of my past life and present circumstances consumed me. I thought about my high school classmates and wondered what they were thinking when they didn't see me in school. I thought about how I would never be able to go back to school and how all the dreams I had of becoming a doctor would never come to pass. I was worried about my three younger sisters and how I always wanted to set a great example for them and wondered if they would ever understand, would they still love me and respect me? The thoughts were endless. I hardly wanted to walk in our neighborhood as I felt so ashamed. Shame and sorrow overwhelmed me.

As the months wore on, the reality that I was really going to have a baby settled in, and my abdomen was growing larger and larger. Finally, in September, my baby son was born. The first few days were extremely difficult as I struggled emotionally to accept my reality; I was so scared and I had no idea how to handle him. My mom was still overseas, but the nurses were very caring and supportive and assisted me tremendously. I remembered the midwife saying to me, "My dear I know it's hard now, but I promise you, you will get through this." I don't think she understood how much her words meant to me, but it was a little ray of hope in a dark pit. I got home with the baby and was grateful I could see my toes standing up and I didn't have what seemed like a barrel in front of me anymore. My mom was now present from the United States and she started showing me how to care for the baby, she was very supportive and that started to give me more hope. Three months later, in December I migrated to the United States with my baby and my mom.

As I settled in, and with my mom helping with the care of the baby, I started inquiring about school and the possibility of getting my high school diploma. I started attending church regularly with my mom and started developing a real relationship with the Lord. I would have regular conversations with the Lord and ask Him to help me. In one year, I was able to get my high school diploma and was accepted into nursing school. Four years later at the age of twenty, I graduated from nursing school as a Registered Nurse in the State of New York. My journey was long and challenging as I battled depression and often cried over the loss of my dad. I cried for the last time on the anniversary of his death ten years later. My healing and restoration came as I spent time with the Lord and opened my heart to His unfailing love, along with Godly counseling. He allowed me to be able to love my son unconditionally and healed my heart of the many wounds I incurred along life's journey. Today, I am a Medical Doctor, along with having three PhDs in Clinical Psychology, Philosophy, and Theology. Today, I have triumphed over the circumstances that were meant to destroy my destiny and render my life useless.

As I look back at my journey, from the loss of my dad suddenly, followed shortly by a horrific assault, I no longer ask, why did this happen to me? The truth is that I now look at what God has brought me through with a grateful heart. Even though I dropped out of high school, I now have four doctoral degrees and an MBA. My son is now a successful accomplished businessman and a Minister. I believe having the support of my mom, godly counseling, and developing a relationship with the Lord allowed me to arise from the ashes of my grief and pain to fulfill my purpose. I am grateful I worship a God who specializes in turning horrible circumstances into platforms of greatness for His glory. I am thankful I have been able to share my story and to be a reference point of hope for many. I have been given platforms to share with women from around the world and to be a source of encouragement to many, letting them know it is possible to overcome your setbacks, your grief, and pain. Look through the lens of gratitude; there's too much to accomplish to wallow in the yesterday of why.

In retrospect, I am thankful that my painful experiences have made me a stronger, more resilient, accomplished individual who can empathize with others experiencing grief and pain. During my journey, it was clear that the life I had planned was not going to happen and definitely not in the order I had planned. Being a mother ushered me into an era of responsibility that I had to own quickly. I also had to develop other important character traits to help get me out of my abyss of shame, low self-esteem, and depression. Another trait I had to develop was confidence. I had to remind myself that my circumstances were not my fault, and as challenging as they were, I could still do something worthwhile with my life. I reminded myself that many had experienced similar atrocities and have managed to overcome them, and by God, I was going to be one of those who rose above the challenges. The next trait I had to develop was perseverance. I had to go back to school and work arduously to accomplish my dreams, and quitting was never going to be an option. No one was going to break me and destroy my destiny.

Today, I am no longer broken, depressed, or filled with pain and shame, but to the contrary, my heart is blazing with joy and the essence of true fulfillment. The sunlight of God's amazing grace has melted away my brokenness and pain like wax melted by the hot sun. In my liberation from the grips of depression and shame, through counseling and God's grace, I now spend a lot of time sharing my story and encouraging broken, wounded souls. In March 2019, I was invited to speak by the United Nations at the 63rd Commission on the Status of Women, addressing issues affecting girls and women globally. I was invited back to the General Assembly of the United Nations in September 2019 to speak on how to empower families. I have traveled to countries including Nigeria and Ghana numerous times, working with abused women and families who are hurting and disenfranchised, giving them a voice and bringing hope to them through various empowerment programs. I have also been sharing with various groups in the United States and Jamaica, encouraging and motivating those who think there's no way out of their pain. Many have been empowered and liberated to shine by God's grace.

As I travel from country to country, I am convinced undoubtedly that there are some things that are common to us as individuals. Our experiences may differ but the truth is, the pain, the hurt, and the disappointment we feel are real. Grief has several different stages and it's important to go through the different stages to emerge on the other side liberated. Getting stuck in any particular stage is unhealthy and prolongs the process. In the throes of depression and grief, living doesn't seem like a great option, but if you can just for a moment stop and look to the One who created you, then there's hope. Going through the process alone is daunting, but professional counseling and divine intervention will interrupt the cycles of mental inertia that seek to keep you bound. Let nothing or no one break you. They didn't make you; you are God's masterpiece. You will get through this!

STEPS TOWARDS INTENTIONAL HEALING

Journeying through grief and pain takes serious work and commitment to not only survive but thrive. Here are a few steps to guide your intentional progress.

- Take responsibility for your outcome. This requires being willing to go through the processes that will lead to healing; Owning the situation and taking responsibility for wanting to get help and following through with the process; Knowing that no one can take responsibility for you.

- Actively participate in your own breakthrough.

- Develop and practice perseverance, self-confidence, and persistence, and adopt a mindset of never ever giving up. This mindset must permeate your being on your way to becoming W.H.O.L.E:

  Wise: The journey to wholeness requires wisdom in every area of your life.

  Healthy: Address your Spiritual, Physical, and Emotional Health. Forgiving yourself and those who hurt you is a critical part of the healing process.

  Organized: Organize your life and your environment, knowing that success favors the prepared.

  Lion-hearted: Be tenacious; relentlessly pursue your freedom and your dreams.

  Evolutionary: Above all else dare to change, to grow, to become the version of you that you aspire to be. Dare to rise from the ashes of your grief, your assault, your loss, your pain, and your disappointment.

Believe in yourself and claim that a new day is dawning in your life. Your Scars will become Stars. Let nothing or no one break you, for they didn't make you. You are God's masterpiece.

RESOURCES

Linktree: www.linktr.ee/drivanahthomas

Instagram: @drivanahthomas

Linkedin: www.inkedin.com/in/ivanah-thomas

CHAPTER 19

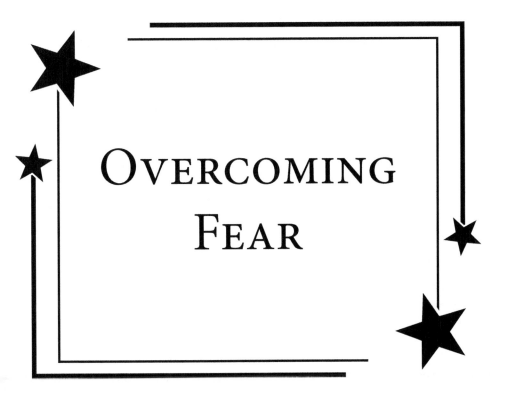

OVERCOMING FEAR

BY: DEBBIE-ANN DYER

DEBBIE-ANN DYER

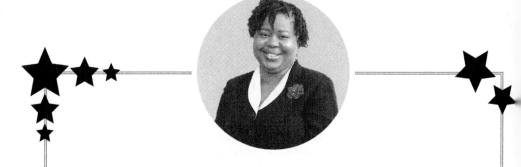

FEAR - Feelings of Excruciating Agony Released
- Dyer (2022)
For God hath not given us the spirit of fear; but of power, and of
love, and of a sound mind. - 2 Timothy 1:7

Debbie-Ann Dyer, a Christian writer and motivational speaker, hails from Williamsfield, situated in North East St. Elizabeth, Jamaica. She has, over the years, enjoyed excellence in academia and has also made her mark in the corporate world. Writing provided the platform on which she stood to herald the truth of God's Word based on her relationship with Him. She continues to fulfill her promise to God to declare His words, as she lay on the side of the road after a terrible accident in December 2002. She remains pliable in the hands of the Master as He creates His masterpiece. Her second book, Spiritual Nuggets: A Sojourner's Insight, was published in 2016 and continues to inspire its readers. Through Her Eyes: A Creative Expression on Relationships through the Eyes of a Christian Woman is a fictional story addressing various social and relational issues within the family construct. It is her hope that it will ignite conversation relating to the relationships we share as Christians and propel us to be deliberate in taking action to make them better. Her latest work as a Intentional Healing: From Scars to Stars contributor is positioned to motivate readers to not allow fear to win.

INTENTION

As you join me on this journey of overcoming fear my hope is that you will see how to deal with fear. Fear has a tendency to repackage itself and attack in various ways; it enjoys being your partner. It is my intention that as you read, you will be able to recognise the presence of fear in your life and the crippling effect it is having or can have. Fear cripples and causes mental turmoil. It is no easy feat to tackle fear, but I assure you that with God's help and continuous effort, you will be like I am. Let us put that demon to shame!

OVERCOMING FEAR

The sun peeped over the horizon, making preparations for its big, bold, and bright arrival. What a beauty! The sky had a picturesque view. The plants rejoiced, the animals awoke, the roosts of the fowls emptied, activities buzzed, and the darkness of night surrendered to the light of day. Morning had come. "Good morning Mommy and Daddy." This was the start of an ordinary day for the Williams family of four at that time.

Mom was the super mom, a loving wife and wonderful homemaker. Looking back now, it would have been good if I stuck to learning how to crochet, knit, or any other skills she tried to teach me, although I think I may have caught a bit of the cooking for she sure knew how to cook. Dad, the rock, was to be feared, but he was the one who had us cracking up with laughter at the games' table and made us appreciate various genres of music. The farmer got us involved on the farm and that was fun. Now I actually like feeling soil through my fingers, watching flowers grow and bloom in season. There is nothing like eating something that you nourished and watered into being.

My sweetheart of a sister was my joy and pain. I could not wrap my head around her inquisitive escapades and her tomboy behaviour; she knew how to get under my skin. I watched her climb the fruit trees and made sure she filled her belly with the delectable fruits while I salivated. There was no way that I was going to climb and the day I decided to follow her step by step to the top of the mango tree, she scaled down and left me begging for help. As for the creepy lizards and frogs, she made it her joy to watch me squirm as she got them to contaminate my skin. But, unacceptable to my parents, she became my punching bag.

At that time, school was great. Basic school was where my ability to do well academically was recognized and the journey to success started. When I got to the age to move on to primary school, it was a no-brainer that I would attend the school where my mother taught. I was usually in the top tier of the class whenever exam results were finalized. I had it going on – bright spark.

It was another normal afternoon. The bell rang for Dick, Rex, and Tarzan to come for dinner, and the rest of the family sat at the table for the sumptuous meal prepared by Mom. However, normalcy suddenly plummeted into horror as political unrest sought to claim its next victims. The raucous outside accompanied by stones pelting through the glass doors and windows threatened our safety. The survival instinct in dad was magnified and he led us on our escape route through the back door, up the hill, through the morass (where we were saved from the suction of the sink hole by other victims already ahead), through the cane fields and finally in the safely of my aunt's home in the neighboring district. But, at six years old my young impressionable mind, like the hot iron frying the label on the skin of cattle, was branded 'FEAR.'

Since then, lost in the abyss of my thoughts, the seed of fear was fertilized with negativity as a defense mechanism. Always prepare for the worst and give thanks if better comes. I have had to grapple with fear clothed in different suits to fit into various areas of my life. In my early years of education, I enjoyed the commendations and being in the top tier of every grade. But, when the result of the national examination used to determine high school was published, my name was not in the papers. The fear of failure punctuated my educational pursuits, for in high school, I had my share of struggles and my progress report after second year in college was stamped discontinued.

Low self-esteem and anger were the results of the fear of not being accepted. I chose to believe the lie that I was ugly. After all, that is what "yuh face big like, yuh lips big like liver and yuh red like malatta" translated to mean. So, if anyone dared to say otherwise, in my mind, they were all liars. That fear made me build a cage around me that even the strongest vice grips or iron cutter would have a hard time breaking.

Fear and anxiety formed an alliance whenever I was in a crowd. As soon as I arrived at an event, I would chart my way of escape because it was guaranteed I would need it later. Blackness beckoned to me in the sunlight as migraines ravished my head. The crowd seemed like vampires determined to suck my blood. The turmoil in my mind, my oozy stomach, and my nerves going haywire were soon evident in the mixture that gushed from my mouth and nostrils.

"What the caterpillar calls the end of the world, the master calls a butterfly." - Richard Bach

Fear is not an easy enemy. But, thank God I met The Master. There is awesome victory when we allow the transformative power of the truth of God's Word to permeate the mind. Believe it! It is very important that my thought life is positive and influenced by the truth of the Word of God. Now I know that fear is not from God (2 Timothy 1:7), so I am very deliberate in using God's word to combat fear. Like the psalmist said, "What time I am afraid, I will trust in thee" (Psalm 56:3, KJV). I have learnt to identify fear and name it for what it is. So, rather than allowing it to sneak into my life and take control, I am now able to nip it in the root.

It is often said and may have been proven that thoughts turn into words which turn into actions, and so I had to retrain my mind and pray that my every thought be brought in captivity to the knowledge of God (2 Corinthians 10:5). It is very important that I guard my mind from the lies of the adversary, so I have a poster with Philippians 4:8 in my bedroom as a constant reminder that my thoughts should be based on truth, that which is honourable, just, pure, lovely and of a good report. I now accept that I am beautiful for that is how God made me (Psalm 139:13-14). Having a good mindset changes the outlook on life.

One of the things that has definitely helped is being in constant prayer and maintaining open communication with God. I recall being challenged by the final exam of Calculus II when pursuing my bachelor's degree. I had a good grade going into the exam but somehow I had a relapse. So, I closed the books after practicing for some pointless hours and poured out my heart in prayer in between sobs in the bathroom. I went to the exam and prayed before the invigilator instructed us to start. I finished the paper in less than half the allotted time, reviewed the paper a few times and handed in the paper. I ended the class with an A. Prayer does help! It is only a pity I did not understand the power of prayer years before when fear captivated me and all I could write on the final exam paper was my name, which along with other factors resulted in a status of discontinued. That label did not stop me from pursuing further studies and graduating with the yellow cord around my neck.

I still have migraines but the trigger is certainly not fear of crowds anymore. The eyes no longer pierce through to my soul, rendering me helpless. I am now very deliberate in identifying the positive in all situations rather than the negative. I now smile from my heart when I look in the mirror for I have redefined the way I see myself. I am beautiful, brilliant, and destined to be greater.

I am thankful for a great support system called family and others that believed in me. As I struggled to get a grip and overcome the challenges I faced in life, my family has been my tower. Despite the failures, they encouraged me and were very active in my moving forward. I have had episodes of setbacks but I confidently declare that "I am no longer a slave to fear."

As we forage through the challenges of life, it is often by default that we ask, why me? Why do I have to go through this? I have had those same experiences, but I have learnt to see the good in life's situations and have been very intentional in seeking to identify the things for which I need to be grateful. My encounters with fear have taught me to be resilient and strong. I am thankful for the determination that was birthed within me. So, I will keep working until the goal is realized.

I have come to recognize that failure does not define me. Although I have failed, I am not a failure. It is simply an experience that will pass and the lessons learnt should be used for the success ahead. I do not measure my worth by people's opinion of me. Rejection, disappointment, and all other negative things serve as fertilizer in the soil ideal for my success.

I have accepted that God's declaration of who I am in Him is the truth by which to live. I am thankful for the person I am now and am looking forward to the person that God is making me become.

As I reminisce on the journeys I have had with fear, I now recognize that I am stronger, more resilient, more determined, and poised to take on new frontiers because of it. Some vital lessons were learnt: never make assumptions about others nor treat anyone with indifference. There are individuals that are battling with some serious issues that have affected them and possibly are being transferred to others, so be more caring. I value the importance of being mindful of other persons' needs and catering to them as best as I can.

Overcoming fear has made me become more brave, daring myself to do that which would have caused me to cower in defeat in time past. So, I have stood before audiences and congregations declaring the word of God and singing to His glory with confidence. Having surrendered to the Master, the caterpillar has morphed into a butterfly with eagle-like characteristics.

I am simply thankful that I am able to function where faith has taken the place of fear. Faith and fear cannot coexist. So, by faith, I will be a bestselling author with a website where I can share the words that I am inspired to write. As I reflected on the various experiences I have had because of fear, I am challenged to write a book. The working title is Unshackled: Feelings of Excruciating Agony Released, publication date to be announced.

I will complete the academic pursuits that I have been procrastinating about for too many years. When my present becomes my past, I will look back and say, "Well done."

Some may give up and throw in the towel. Others may die, although they live, as fear grips. But, faith and fear cannot coexist, so choose to exercise faith. Be determined to push against the odds. The tide may be going in the opposite direction, but swim against the tide. Cut against the grain. Do not allow fear to prevent you from realizing your goals. Do not allow fear to rob you of a fulfilled and happy life. Do not allow fear to hinder you from living in your purpose.

The victory at Jericho was after thirteen marches around the wall (Judges 5). Naaman had to dip into Jordan seven times before he experienced healing (2 Kings 5). You have overcome other challenges in life and you can certainly overcome this one. It is time to do that thing again. Go back to school. Write that book. Forgive that friend. This time may be the charm!

Steps Towards Intentional Healing

Recently, I was sharing at the book club that I am a part of and I said, "God knows the plans He has for us, but we have to be active players for the plans to be realized." Therefore, I recommend these three steps as you seek to heal intentionally and navigate from scars to stars:

Develop and maintain a relationship with God. This will allow you to have clarity on what to do and our need to be obedient. It is without apology that I declare you nor I could not be here without God. So, have an active prayer life, study and apply the word of God to your life, and ensure that dependence is on God and not self.

Be intentional about being thankful. This has the potential to result in a shift of focus from the effects of fear and all the wrong things to that which you should and can be thankful for. So, start a thankfulness journal. At the end of each day or week, reflect on the things for which you are thankful. This may help you realize that there are some things that are a part of daily life that are taken for granted. It may make you come to terms with the fact that even though life is not what you would want it to be, it could be worse, so appreciate every moment and experience for what it is worth.

Engage in self-development activities. Instead of being held captive by fear, get involved in those things that will improve your life spiritually, educationally, physically, emotionally and in other "allys." Find a hobby or skill that you enjoy. Do that thing that you have been procrastinating about for too long, like go back to school, love again, write the book, learn to knit; just do that thing you have always wanted to do.

Resources

Facebook: https://www.facebook.com/debbieann.dyer

Instagram: https://instagram.com/debbieannwdyer

Tiktok: https://www.tiktok.com/@d.ann.dyer

CHAPTER 20

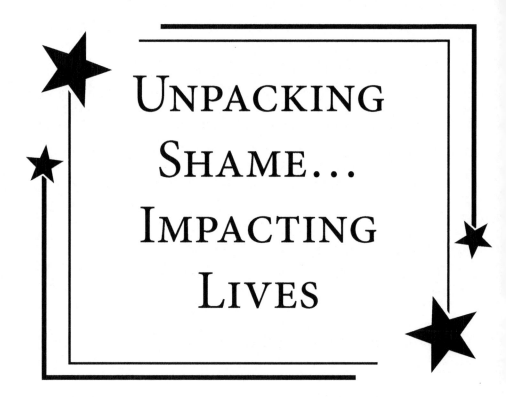

UNPACKING
SHAME...
IMPACTING
LIVES

BY: ELAINE OXAMENDI VICET

ELAINE OXAMENDI VICET

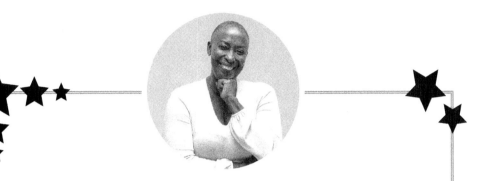

"I can always better, my best."

Elaine Oxamendi Vicet is a nurturer; a developer of talent and random acts of kindness are akin to the essence of her spirit and existence. She naturally bursts into a smile and is the first to see solutions rather than sight the problems. She is a speaker of truth with a diplomatic flair, an accomplished writer and poet, and has co-authored a textbook and a children's book. Some of Elaine's works have been deposited with the National Library of Jamaica. Unabashed to share her story, Elaine has spoken to young women at a number of forums where she talks openly of her experience and the need to forgive oneself. Whether in a group or sharing one-on-one, Elaine reminds people that holding on to shame is a choice even when something shameful happens. A peacekeeper, Elaine is an active member of the Justices of the Peace of Jamaica, Kingston.

INTENTION

You will journey with the author from her fledgling years when she was introduced to unwanted touch. Trust became an issue for her; although hidden from everyone, she learned to masquerade her pain and shame. Constantly failing at love, she journeys overseas leaving all that she knew. One day, she answered the door and had a life-changing experience. Years later, having "kissed a few frogs" her prayer is finally answered. Within ten weeks of meeting her Romeo, she weds and casts caution to the wind. Despite his love and support, she still struggles to unpack her childhood shame.

UNPACKING SHAME...IMPACTING LIVES

It was the cusp of the 1970s, and there was always talk from my parents of ways of keeping us safe. There were four of us from this union with two from previous marriages on the maternal side. It was a loving and caring family where the boys were told to take care of the girls. It was their responsibility to keep the girls safe.

Life as a child in this house of six and occasional family members, visiting or short-term living arrangements was fun. Sundays were for the family, as we would go on "drive-outs" and buy takeout or just drive and explore new places.

On returning home, my mother always had a dessert ready to be placed on the table. Simply yummy moments as we sat together as a family, my father would share stories as we listened.

My sister and I had our own fantasy world and assigned ourselves alien characters, made up our own language that sounded like "Ku-Ku-

Kum-Kuh." We totally understood each other. More of a tomboy myself, I climbed trees and would swing from any tree whether it was the cotton tree, grapefruit, apple, or even the coconut tree.

Safety was a premium. So, perimeter fences of privet and barbed wire were removed and upgraded to nine-foot concrete walls. The entire house was grilled. We never feared for anything, only those characters from the tales my mother told: the proverbial 'Blackheart' man, 'mancod,' and 'rolling calf. A rule-based house was what we knew. My father was a stern man, he was the wielder of discipline, but what was worse were those long talks when there was an infraction after the whooping and tears. In spite of it, we felt loved and protected, and growing up was fun.

My parents, having fortified the yard, turned their attention to making the play space safe. Men were hired to make the flooring of the now grilled patio safe for play. We were cautioned to stay inside while the men were at work. But I was curious, so I watched the patio transform.

The contractor called out to me and asked me for "cream." I thought he meant "ice cream." And so I asked my mother, and she said, "He meant hand lotion," which is what he calls "cream."

Bright-eyed and innocent, I took the bottle and carefully handed it to him; at under five feet and less than fifty pounds, he pulled me in and shoved his adult tongue in my mouth. I gasped, pulled away, and ran inside leaving my small footprint in the green-tiled concrete.

How could I tell my father? Best not to say anything. I know my father may do this man grave harm; best not to tell him.

I retreated and kept my secret and shame safe.

My mother, I thought, somehow suspected something but she never said anything to me. Perhaps she, from the "old school," didn't know what to say or how.

Bright-eyed and naïve, a few years later, a family member took advantage of me for what felt like forever. Naïve and silly, I innocently reported daily for the abuse not knowing it to be wrong. Just shy of going the full distance, my mother intervened and put an end to the daily treks to the forbidden space.

She never told my father. The risk was great and my mother took the line of least resistance and simply forbade me from going to that space.

Later, I came to learn that it was terribly wrong and in sharing with some female family members, they too revealed a similar experience. It certainly couldn't get any worse but life was about to go into a tailspin.

Not barely twelve, an adolescent girl was allowed to stay over. She was from the same church; being an orphan, my parents, having big hearts allowed her to stay with us.

At nights, in the same bed, there would be unwanted touches. How could I tell? I was suffering abuse yet again.

The shame and this shameful experience dug deep in my skin. How could I trust anyone? Who could make me feel secure; when and how would I ever be safe?

I learned Taekwondo and built muscles. I proposed that no one would take advantage of me. I removed the scales from my eyes and saw men and women as they are. I learned to profile persons quickly and forged my armour early. I was taking matters into my own hands.

Never would I let my guard down and never would I let anyone touch me unless I wanted them to. It was now my turn.

So it was just going to be me and me alone. I had to keep myself strong and safe.

I was never able to maintain a successful relationship; whenever it moved from fledging to something serious, I found a way to destroy and decimate it, one failed relationship after another. I reconciled that I would never wed; never be happy; never find anyone who could forgive me of my childhood shame.

All that time, I was looking in the wrong direction. I went to church every Sunday but I never knew God. I never met Christ, so I tumbled and rolled. I trusted no one and hid my shameful experience from everyone. My twenties rolled by and I now lived in a foreign land. I had no care in the world as I worked and lived for fun. Why not?! You live only once. But that was not how God planned it.

I remember that day as if it was yesterday. The day when I answered the call and my scars were removed and finally, I could hold my head up and look to the stars.

There was a knock on the door at the house where I lived. I opened and there stood two bible-toting ladies, smiling. I welcomed them and they shared their story and journey to "Christ the King." I listened. I knew my soul was ready.

I was so weighed down and released all at the same time as I listened to them. When they left, I went to my room, knelt in my bed, sobbed, and bawled out for forgiveness. I sobbed and prayed. I asked the Lord Jesus to enter my life and in that moment I was saved. My catharsis had begun. I felt safe for the first time, safe and redeemed.

Since the shameful experiences, I had done it my way and I learned to make myself physically strong and kept myself safe by learning self-defence; I gave myself a new start by journeying overseas but with all that, God said not my way but His.

Safe and free, I could go home.

Home. I knew the Lord. He had my back. He kept me. Bible study empowered me and I was well on my way. I was garnering the tools to unpack my shame and felt comfortable telling my story. Yes, finally after so many burdened years, I could tell all the details. In a face-to-face, one-on-one, or group session or just saying it to my friends or family, I could unpack my shame and share the tools that led me to feel safe.

Over the years, I learned different ways to express gratitude and just be grateful. I grew in gratitude for small acts of kindness, be it someone just listening to me or saying "I love you," I always say, "Thank you." I do not take it for granted that I am loved.

I am grateful for waking. Thank you Lord for waking me up, I do not take it for granted that I lived to see this day, and so I say thank you for this first gift called life. My prayer each morning is one of thanks.

I am grateful that I view my shame experiences as lessons learnt that I can use to improve my life and that of some others.

I remain grateful that God prepared me for whirlwind love for ten weeks before getting married; we are now living in our two-plus decades of marriage.

I remain grateful as I reconciled the chink in my life. I learned how to forgive myself, as that had always been my stumbling block, not feeling worthy and feeling vulnerable.

I am grateful I learnt to forgive.

I learnt tolerance, trust, humility, and ownership.

Going through my catharsis is a daily walk. My character is continuously being refined.

I have grown more tolerant of people who are dogmatic and I suspect less of the motives of people. I have learned not to figure out why someone says or does something. Over the years, I simply learned to apply the Johari Window when dealing with people.

I am now more trusting of others, as I learn to unpack my story and share it as lessons learnt, thereby creating a testimony, realising that I am better today than I was yesterday.

I learned to be humble and treat each experience as valuable, regardless of who is saying or doing; I can learn from that person.

I have learnt that I can own my experiences without being ashamed of those experiences. I have learned that bad things can happen; however, the fact that they happen does not make me a bad person or unworthy. I have learned that the biggest gift is to forgive yourself.

I have learned to accept my vulnerability and moments of insecurity. I have learned to take ownership of my pain and shame. With acceptance and ownership, I heal.

The thing is, I have found over the years that my relationship with the Lord is empowering. Letting go of shame and accepting the experience as a lesson is also empowering. Owning my vulnerability and daring to share and tell my story have empowered me and others as they also grow and release their own shame.

I focus a lot on my relationship with the Lord. I trust the Lord. It doesn't always feel as if He has my back, even though I know He always does. It is that awareness that there is a higher power, my Creator who is taking me through it all. I love the story as it is told in Matthew 14:22-33; Peter needed only to stay focused on the Lord and not allow the torment to distract him. Yet as he was sinking, Christ was only an arm's reach away. I am encouraged by that and keep it close to me; so much so, that it defines me and empowers me and I use it to empower and encourage others.

I kept my secret for years. Scarred and jaded, I recluded. I know now that not telling was bad.

Every day I unpack and strip away another layer. I tell my story without feeling shame and in doing so, I heal. I learn from year to year that FORGIVENESS really is a BIG THING. When the Lord says I am FORGIVEN, it is just that!

It is not easy. It takes a constant reminder…self to self…that there is no shame in having had a shameful experience; even if I were the cause of it…even if I was careless…even if others took advantage…I still remain FORGIVEN.

Step by step, I begin each day with gratitude for the opportunity to share with others. It is never over until God says so. I have forgiven that man; I remember his face, and I forgive him. I forgive that girl; I remember her name, and I forgive her. I have forgiven my family member, and I forgive him. And I forgive myself for ever thinking that I was at fault and that I was condemned for those shameful experiences.

I just forgive!

STEPS TOWARDS INTENTIONAL HEALING

As you also seek to heal intentionally and move from scars to stars, here are three things that resonate:

I am forgiven! It is really important to realise forgiveness is a truism. Forgiveness of self is a life imperative. It is the first step to healing.

Second, it is important to own the pain and shame. Learning to accept and own the pain and shame of whatever experience that occurred is part of life. It may not be the best of experiences all the time... but when we get knocked down, we get up and tell, tell, just tell the story to someone. By telling and getting up, we are made stronger and more resilient. Get up! Tell others and they will help you to stand and heal!

Finally, choosing how to respond to an experience is a choice. One can choose to feel shame and carry it and let it colour life's experiences and prevent the formation of better experiences. Or the choice can be made to use the experience and positively learn from it. In learning from it, we share and help others. A selfless act is an act of kindness; it is prescriptive and healing. Helping others to unpack their shame is tantamount to saving lives!

RESOURCES

Instagram: @elainevicet

Facebook: Elaine Oxamendi Vicet

LinkedIn: Elaine Oxamendi Vicet

CHAPTER 21

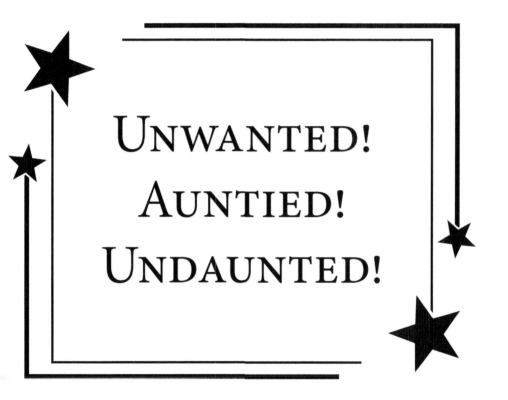

UNWANTED! AUNTIED! UNDAUNTED!

BY: RAYMOND NELSON

RAYMOND NELSON

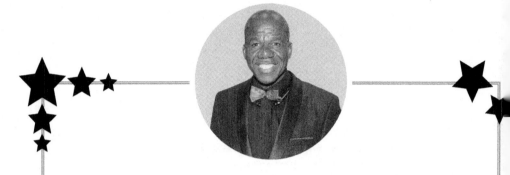

Every time I remember to forget, it makes forgiveness harder yet!
- Ray Nelson (2022)

Singer, poet, comedian, businessman, and a Master of Ceremonies, Raymond "Nello" Nelson was often told by his teachers that he was a joker, so he did not disappoint them. He attributes his sense of humor and comedic skills to growing up with seven siblings. Backyard concerts with each child performing at his mother, Normsie's, house resulted in plenty of laughter to go around.

His grandfather, DJ Murphy, worked at the Bellevue Mental Hospital in Jamaica until his retirement, so there were lots of stories. His father owned a furniture factory off Woodpecker Avenue in Kingston, Jamaica, and there was lots of drama among the workers. When he was around 11 years old, his parents moved the family to Waltham Park Road with the hopes of providing a better social environment for the children. Ironically, the house was next to two rum bars and a betting shop so there were lots of prayers.

Ray believes that laughter can be found in every situation.

A graduate of Northern Caribbean University (NCU), formerly West Indies College in Mandeville Jamaica and Baruch College (CUNY), in New York, he holds degrees in Business and International Marketing respectively.

He currently lives in the United States, where he owns and manages Double Line Auto in Hampton, New Jersey.

INTENTION

Have you ever gone through something so painful that you don't want to share it with anyone because it might put a thought in their head…a thought that was never there before? The fact of the matter is that you are so fearful that they might end up thinking the same thing about you that you were scared to share with them in the first place. As you journey with me, you will experience how being teased and called names can be devastating. You will learn that even fear, compounded fear, can be overcome.

UNWANTED! AUNTIED! UNDAUNTED!

I grew up in a family of eight children, four boys and four girls—and we loved each other dearly. We teased each other, we bantered with each other, we just had fun with each other, but we never used hurtful nicknames. More often than not, our nicknames were just shortened versions of our real names. For Cecilia, it was Cecile, Beverly was Bev, Michael was Mike or Junior, Patrick was just Patrick, Joan was just Joan; Janet was Janet, Richmond was Richie, and Raymond was Rayie. There were eight of us going around having fun. As children we would entertain ourselves; we did not need others from outside to help us have fun. We had some friends with similar backgrounds—they came from large families like us who would come over and we would enjoy ourselves. But as we got older and went to different schools, we would tease a little and get a little teasing too; that was just normal. We were able to give-and-take, but some names you just brushed it off while others stuck to you. They would give you a short affectionate name for your last name: for Brown it would be Brownie, for Nelson it was like Nello or, as one guy called me, Nellie Oleson, which was from the Little House on the Prairie Television series. So, they started calling me Nellie and then it became Nello….thank goodness it evolved to Nello! These AKAs are called terms of endearment and can follow you for the rest of your life (even now, friends I grew up with still call me Nello).

Richmond and Raymond. Raymond and Richmond. We were inseparable, and no one could get it right…although we do not look or sound alike. We were like twins; we never even knew that we looked differently, although I was darker skin tone than he was. Richmond and Raymond…. twins. Although my brother was one year older than me, everyone treated us like twins; they would ask us which one is older. We got in trouble together, got spanked together, got treats together, and did everything together. Richmond and Raymond, Raymond and Richmond. It was easier just to call us together, so that's what everyone in the family did…. Richmond and Raymond stood together like one name. Life was simple. Life was good. Why can't we just be cowboys again? Howdy Partner!

My father would bring my uppity grand-aunt to visit us once in a while. On one of these visits, she called me by mistake; she said, "Raymond come here," and I came as fast as I could. "Yes Auntie." She said, "Not you. I was calling the handsome one. Where is he?" I thought to myself, as I came to a screeching halt (and so did my then perfect world), "Okay you must probably mean Richmond." Salt was added to my wound as I was tasked with going to get my brother, Richmond. Now, do you know how that affected me for the rest of my life? It did not create any jealousy because we were brothers; we just were brothers. We did not look at each other as good or "gooder" looking; we were just cowboys… the good, the bad, and the sometimes-ugly duo. We just looked at each other as brothers. We fought and played and had good times. Why can't we be cowboys again?

At that point in life, I was becoming more aware of my surroundings, and my confidence was shaken by what my aunt did. She couldn't take it back, I know, but she never apologized. She never tried to even make it up to me….she could very easily have bribed me with a little ice cream or something sweet. Was she aware of the damage she caused? Maybe not. However, I think my dad told her because every time he tried to take me to her house, I refused and reminded him that I am not going "because I'm not the handsome one." He always replied with, "We must learn to forgive." Yes, I did forgive, but at 10 years old, forgiveness was not something I could process extensively. The words my aunt used were indelibly etched on my mind. You can't seem to take it back; it was painful because I lived with that, and I didn't say anything much about it. Sometimes, my siblings would try to dismiss it and say, "Ah Ray, come on man..." Yes, that might seem okay to some people but for me it was not okay. Now that my eyes are sensitive to prejudices, injustices, and double standards, it did not jive with me. I'm very aware that this happens with families and other people. Now, it makes me an advocate for those who I see treated as the underdogs.

I am not in a crisis mode! I don't have identity, abandonment, or self-esteem issues. But, I do have issues accepting the fact that I may have had all these issues at some point in my life.

Every time I hear people say, "Oh, the baby was ugly," or something like that, I get up and try to leave the room and I tell them there is no such thing as an ugly baby. I want to bring something that affected me to your attention.

I tried, I really tried. I pressed delete. I hit delete. But, it will not delete. The data was bad! It stuck like glue. I pressed delete but still nothing new.

Let me tell you when the spell broke. The spell broke many years later, probably about twenty years ago while I was at a car auction. The auctioneer was trying to get my attention to purchase a car and he said, "You, you over there—Denzel, Denzel Washington." I looked up and he said, "Yeah, you!" And I thought to myself, "Wow!" At that moment, I realized that if I even remotely looked like Denzel Washington—even to this white guy who probably does not know how to differentiate one Black person from another—then there must be something about how I looked. I wore that on my sleeve, and I took on that new feature, like Yeah! Oh, I forgot to tell you that I was always known as a great dresser. Why did I dress very well? Maybe because I wanted to be noticed as a good dresser. My fashion sense was impeccable, even though I didn't have a big wardrobe, and it was evident to everyone by the way I dressed and carried myself that I took a lot of pride in myself.

I also realized that sometimes we compensate or overcompensate to get past situations in our lives or overcome something that we are enduring. But after that as I read the Bible and read again the story about Rachel and Leah, Esau and Jacob, Martha and Mary, Joseph and his brothers, and so many more stories that should serve to encourage us to trust again, I realized that they faced similar issues.

I became a giver. I would just give, give, and give, not trying to buy friendships, but to win over hearts, true hearts to myself and my causes. I would show up at times when you would least expect because the Holy Spirit works that way in directing me to fulfill a need; and when there's a need, I see it as my duty to assist in fulfilling it. I consider myself to be very resourceful. I network and connect with persons who can give and others who I can inspire to give all because of what my aunt said to me.

As I sought acceptance and approval from my community, family, and friends, I found new and innovative ways to satisfy my need to succeed. Why do I work so hard? What am I trying to prove? I work hard to ensure that nobody could truly say that I am not deserving of everything that I have achieved in life. There really is no free lunch. The respect I receive and the rewards are commensurate with my efforts. Now, I live a life that is more qualitative than quantitative, and relationships have become my priority.

By writing poetry, I have found a way to release my "penned up" thoughts and emotions as well as to express myself through the eyes of different individuals.

Finally, I became intentional in moving beyond my grief. I was among a group of persons who went through Dr. Grace Kelly's "21 Day Plan for Personal Grieving, Healing, and Restoration" program. We were often reminded by her that "pain not identified cannot be healed." I completely agreed with that and addressed many of the issues I wrote about in this chapter as suggested by the contents of her book Grieve If You Must. I used and continue to use it as a guide to treat my scars.

Not knowing where a person is coming from when they make negative comments can be a trigger for me as it can inflame my old scars. However, my mantra has become "Do unto others as you would like them to do unto you," as found in Matthew 7:12 (KJV). I have learned to be more sensitive, trusting, accepting, resilient, patient, and a little more forgiving. The main character development components for me spell STAR:

INTENTIONAL HEALING: FROM SCARS TO STARS

Sensitivity: I developed a deep feeling for others. I empathize and sympathize with them and assist them in addressing their needs.

Trust: I learned to feel alive again like a little child in a safe place.

Acceptance: I realized that we do not have control over another person's opinion. I also accepted the reality of my situation without complaining or resenting, and instead devised ways to heal my scars.

Resilience: Find and embrace positive feedback in order to override negative data quickly.

I am drawn towards young people who are at a disadvantage because of emotional deficiency due to negative exposures. The love and patience I demonstrated towards my three daughters, I am now seeing expressed by them through their ability to love, especially those who encounter bias, prejudice, or some other types of disenfranchisement. I was intentional in being equally caring and loving toward them and they too have become very, very caring. The memory of being disenfranchised in my early years is now appreciated as it is the foundation of my legacy.

As early as age sixteen, I realized that I was drawn to books like Norman Vincent Peale's The Power of Positive Thinking and Maxwell Maltz's Psycho-Cybernetics. I have now come to realize that I was searching for answers to my scars, even as a teenager. I am very grateful for this opportunity to express how I have navigated MY SCARS to become the shining star I was created to be. My scars surround issues over which I had no control: the size of my nose, my big head, and my knock-knees.

I am an overcomer and I let nothing keep me from being authentic and being true to myself. I no longer self-sabotage by internalizing all the negative things I heard about myself growing up, always thinking that I am "less than." I AM ACTUALIZED. My scars have motivated me towards excellence in everything I do. I discovered that the world actually values skill sets over physical features. Think about it. My negative mindset affected my marriages, my family relationships, my job performance, my social interactions, among other things. I now let people discover who I am and my innate abilities as opposed to my features. If a lady gravitates to me and says, "Hi handsome," or, "I love you," I now trust that they see something in me, not just my physical features. I am now confident that my attributes are beyond my physiology and what others can see, feel, or experience. I know that I am more than a conqueror. I am an overcomer and I can healthily appreciate the person I have become. My scars have shaped me into a star.

Today, I am reaching out to you to let you see that just as I have overcome my scars, you can too. This is what I now do to shine: I advocate for persons with similar experiences. I am convinced that parents, guardians, and the extended family need to be made aware of these matters. Instead of allowing persons who think that they have a right or a license to verbally abuse our children, parents and the village-at-large need to confront, defend, and promote the rights of that child and their future. This is how we create a healthy emotional environment. These are discussions we need to have openly.

To this end, I advocate in creating awareness for this issue among the village through my writings, poetry, devotionals, humor, and my testimony. Within the next few months, a book of poetry that speaks to real-life situations and captures the emotions of individuals having similar experiences will be released. I endeavor for this chapter in the book, Intentional Healing: From Scars to Stars, to be developed into a complete book. I will also be hosting, collaborating, and sharing my story to various groups through podcasts and other social media avenues.

When parents protect their children early on, children will feel loved and protected.

Sometimes, our parents need to confront and defend and let others know that this is my child you are talking about…be very careful. I am sure if my mom knew about my aunt, she would have kissed it away, yes; she would have hugged me and kissed me on my forehead and that would have helped. My dad probably let it slide thinking I would heal and grow from it. But for a child, that did not happen. When you are feeling "less than," the Holy Spirit will help you make up the difference and THAT can become your calling. So, instead of trying to blame anyone, let us realize that sometimes life chooses us to be the one, even if by default. We need to be positive and be the "chosen one." If you are truly anointed and appointed to a cause, you will receive the gifts needed to answer and fulfill it.

Steps Towards Intentional Healing

I am pleased to offer my acronym **STAR ACT** to help you on your journey towards intentional healing.

Sensitivity: Seek to develop a deep feeling for others and sympathy for their needs regardless of their situation. Always put safety first. Protect yourself from abusive relationships.

Trust: Learn to trust yourself and feel alive again like a little child. Find your safe place.

Acceptance: Realize that we do not have control over another person's opinion or their actions. Accept the reality of your situation without complaining or resenting. Create a plan to navigate through life positively.

Resilience: Being resilient is allowing yourself to be an active participant in your grief. Find and embrace positive thoughts and feedback in order to override negative data quickly.

Acknowledge: Once you are able to identify and acknowledge the source of your pain, you can then take corrective measures to address it.

Confront. After acknowledging your pain, you should confront the issues and work towards controlling your emotions and your triggers.

Talk. Now that you have begun to control your emotions, you will be in a better position to talk about it. This should be your resolution….TO TALK ABOUT IT. Once you can talk about it, you will be able to fix it.

Resources

Linkedin: https://www.linkedin.com/in/ray-nelson-3330a152/

Instagram: https://www.instagram.com/ray_nelson_double_line_auto

Facebook: https://www.facebook.com/ray.nelson.9275

CHAPTER 22

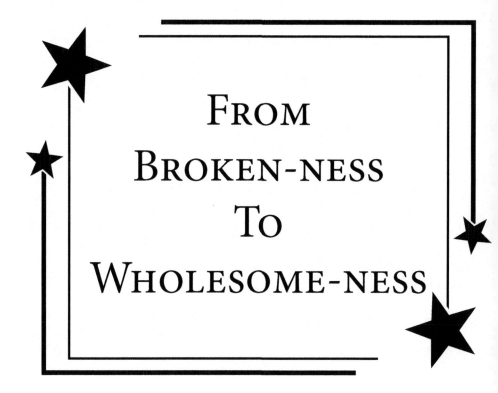

FROM BROKEN-NESS TO WHOLESOME-NESS

BY: DAWN 'LADY D' SAMUELS

Dawn 'Lady D' Samuels

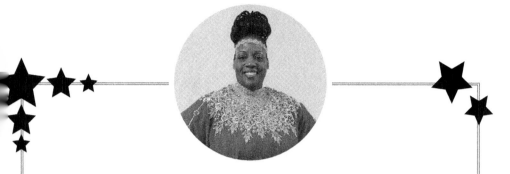

I played no part in the selection of my parents, birth, or how I was raised. Even if I could, I would not change anything.
"Before I formed you, I knew you, and before you were born, I consecrated you; I appointed you a prophet to the nations."
- Jeremiah 1:5 (KJV)

Dawn 'Lady D' Samuels is a native of Jamaica who resides in the borough of the Bronx, NY. She attended Ruseas High, West Indies College High, Northern Caribbean University (formerly West Indies College), Charmaine School of Nursing, Connecticut School of Broadcasting, and Andersonville Theological Seminary where she holds a Bachelor's Degree in Theology. She is a former Radio Broadcaster of Hot 102 Radio in Jamaica, WAVS in Florida and WRTN in New Rochelle, NY. Lady D is presently an international singing/ preaching evangelist, a Gospel recording artist, a Christian comedian, and well sought after emcee. She ministers extensively across the United States, Jamaica WI, Grand Cayman, Grenada, Canada, and the United Kingdom. In 2014, she published her autobiography entitled Alone in a Crowd...from Broken-ness to Wholesome-ness, adding author to her God-given gifts.

She is writing her second book, How I Got Over. She says her greatest accomplishment is raising her two sons, Vynce and BJ. Lady D has dedicated her life to the service of Kingdom building, lifting up the name of Jesus while bringing joy to the brokenhearted and peace to the downtrodden. Her personal mantra is as follows: if you can use anything Lord, you can use me.

INTENTION

I want my readers to know that the beauty and impact of their story is not necessarily in the start but in the outcome. It is not what happens to you that defines you, but it's your response to it and who you are because of the experience. The brightest creations are often birthed out of difficult situations. Like with the evolution of a beautiful piece of diamond, there must be a process of refining, though it's usually uncomfortable and most times painful; the joy and contentment that the final product brings and the light that it creates will illuminate the path for others to follow.

FROM BROKEN-NESS
TO WHOLESOME-NESS

Life became great for a dressmaker in her late 30's who could not fulfill the most important request from her husband. The situation was much like Hannah in the Bible who was praying for a baby for many years. One morning, a single unwed mother showed up at her door and asked her if she could care for her sick child for just one day. Little did the dressmaker know that this was the day for answered prayers. She gave the baby the best care she could. At the end of the day when the mother returned, the dressmaker asked the mother a question that would change the course of many lives including mine. "Can I have her?" "Yes", came the reply. This saga gave birth to my adoption and me having a mama and a daddy.

Life became great for my biological mother as well; she was now able to continue to work and take care of her other children without worrying about caring for a sick child. Later on in life, I would learn of my sickness taking a turn for the worse, how the doctors gave me up for dead, and how a grave spot was selected for my burial. Had it not been for Mama's prayers and the miraculous healing powers of Jehovah Rapha, I would not be alive to tell of the goodness of God.

However, life was good as I grew. I was enrolled in a Seventh Day Adventist private school and was the best-dressed little girl among my peers thanks to Mama's unmatched skills in the field of dressmaking.

I was told that I started singing as soon as I started talking and was dubbed a songbird in my church, school, and community, always entertaining others either by making them laugh from my vast repertoire of jokes or from asking to sing a song for them.

I loved Mama and Daddy and enjoyed spending time with them. Mama was beautiful with long black hair; even at home, she was dressed like she was ready to step out of the house at any given moment. I was fascinated with her strong soprano voice as she belted out notes in the choir at church.

Daddy was of a dark complexion, tall and stately; he captured the attention of everyone when he entered a room. I often waited for Daddy's return from work and would run into his arms with the biggest grin and warmest embrace any little girl can bestow on a father.

Like a deflated balloon, the air was slowly escaping from the life of this happy-go-lucky six-year-old girl. Soon, instead of laughter and singing, there was silence and sadness.

"Joy," (my pet name), "there is something that your father and I want to tell you. We are not your real parents and your name is not Joy Smith. We wanted you to know before anyone else tells you."

They were definitely not prepared for the reaction when I threw myself on the ground and cried for hours screaming that one "pickney" can't have two mothers; I didn"t want anyone else to be my parents. I refused to eat or play and the unhappiness dragged on for days.

This was the beginning of my feelings of rejection. This situation worsened when I met my biological mother and learned that my name, Dawn Samuels, was just a name but I was not related to anyone by the name of Samuels.

Where did the name Samuels come from and who is my father?
INTENTIONAL HEALING: FROM SCARS TO STARS

When I was old enough to understand, I was told that the man Samuels, whose name I carried, was the father of three of my older siblings but was living abroad during the time of my conception and birth, making it impossible for him to carry out the role of a father.

Added to the rejection I felt was now the feeling of abandonment. I felt abandoned by my biological father whom, to date, I still have not met. I also felt abandoned and unloved by my biological mother when I discovered that I had siblings. My young mind could not comprehend why I was given away and the others were not.

I didn't understand that God was setting me up for greatness, taking me through the refining fire. I spent many days in isolation underneath the bed which had become my safe haven. At about age ten, Daddy stopped going to church and started beating Mama severely. Mama and I moved to a different Parish to escape the beatings.

One day, Daddy came to the new location. Mama was not home, so he kicked the door open, stripped the bed of the linen, stripped me of all my clothes, took off his belt, and gave me a beating I will never forget. He said, "As long as you live, don't ever call me Daddy; I am not your father."

That marked the beginning of mistrust and broken relationships.

During the early 1990s, I was a radio broadcaster at Hot 102 Radio in Jamaica and a cabaret artist, performing in various hotels along the North Coast along with my job at the nightclub. As usual I was bringing joy and happiness to others while experiencing a deep deficit of the same.

I had enough money to live a comfortable life, but I was a woman most miserable.

I remember quite vividly leaving the stage, rushing to my hotel room, locking the door behind me, and crying so hard until my body shivered profusely. I remember turning off the "On Air" microphone at work and getting a quick cry before going back on air in a bid to use my tears to wash away the emptiness and loneliness in my heart.

It was during these dark days that I met a former broadcaster in the person of Carlington Sinclair. He was very impressed with my voice and the persona I brought to broadcasting. In one of our conversations, I told him that I didn't feel the way I looked or sounded; I confessed my constant thoughts of suicide, which came as a total shock to him.

He talked to me about the power of affirmation and thought control. He encouraged me to take control of my thoughts by repeating words of affirmation. He encouraged me to write lines of positive affirmations and say them out loud before going to sleep. I was grateful for his advice but was not consistent with its application.

In one of her famous quotes, bestselling author Heather Ash Amara says, "Change is inevitable but transformation is by conscious choice."

My journey from scars to star started years later when I got tired of being sad, miserable, and defeated; I was tired of harboring suicidal thoughts. I knew there must be more to life than this. As I ministered, I longed to experience the happiness and joy that I see on the faces of the people I entertain.

So I made the conscious decision to do something about it.

Remembering the advice I received from my friend many years ago about the power of affirmation, one of the first things I did was to make a chart with my picture in the center making "I am" statements. I wrote as many "I am's" as possible: for example, I am beautiful, I am happy, I am loved, I am accepted, etc.

The next conscious decision I made was to listen to motivational speakers. I started taking notes and tried to apply them to my life. This became a major part of my life. I was hungry as the famous Les Brown would say. I was prepared for the challenge.

Some of my favorites were Les Brown, Bishop TD Jakes, and Pastor Joel Osteen. One day while listening to Joel Osteen, I heard him say that happiness is a choice; we are capable of switching off negative thoughts and choosing our own happiness. I felt like he was speaking directly to me, so that day I made the decision to choose happiness.

I began monitoring the things I listen to, the thoughts I harbored, the television programs I watched, and the people I listened to.

To this day, I only allow myself to watch five minutes of news and avoid things and people who challenge my happiness.

My transformation was not an easy feat; I had to be intentional and worked at it daily, but once I started applying these principles to my life, the scars kept falling off and a light started shining through me.

Many times throughout my early childhood and even as a young adult, I repeatedly asked questions. Why did my mother give me away? Why do I have the name of a man who is not my father? Why did my father forsake me? Who is my father?

As the scars fell off and I realized that my entire existence is for the purpose of service to God and my fellow men, my why me became why not me.

I am grateful I was adopted into a Christian home where I learned about God at an early age. I am grateful for a loving Christian woman who so unselfishly showed me love like I was her own and taught me how to love others. I am grateful for the sickness God brought me through, the grave spot chosen for me was not mine, and because the twists and turns in my life have taken me to where I am today.

As a Minister of the Gospel of Christ, I am given the opportunity to share my story and empower others. When I pray with and encourage others, I can inspire with empathy because I've been there.

There was a time that I yearned for acceptance, always feeling rejected, unworthy, and unloved. Today, my heart is filled with gratitude, knowing that God has chosen me and loves me unconditionally, that I was bought with a price, chosen even before I was born. I now have a sense of belonging. I am no longer feeling like a castaway. I am a blood washed beauty living my divine purpose.

Many studies in the last 40 years indicate that the way we see ourselves determines to a large degree the way we act and react in life. Self-worth and self-esteem tend to be governing factors in our lives.

Many times people ask me how I got from being suicidal to the happy person I am today. I would say it's because my character was developed through my pain. My self-worth has changed.

Knowing who I am has raised my self-esteem, transforming me from nothing to something special, from rejection to acceptance.

Through my struggles, I have become a strong, confident woman of God, capable of giving and receiving love. No longer do I crave the validation of men. I have a father who is crazy about me and that gives me strength. The emptiness is now filled with a tremendous amount of peace and contentment and all my praise belongs to God.

According to John Lederach, "Voice centers upon inclusive conversations that are grounded in mutuality, understanding and accessibility. When individuals have a voice, their views, thoughts, and feelings receive a fair hearing that is readily recognized by others. They possess the ability to influence outcomes and manipulate contexts with words they speak."

From early years, I have been complimented on my voice, the richness of its tone, and my ability to use it effectively to command the attention of others.

My voice is a direct gift from God. It has allowed me to win several speech competitions, elocution contests, and music awards. In later years, it afforded me a place in radio broadcasting.

The Bible says your gifts will bring you before great men. Through the gift of voice, I have been blessed to preach, emcee, and sing to several audiences in many places as I share my story.

Moving forward, I desire to continue to use my story as a conduit, pointing men and women to the God who never fails. I will finish my second book by the end of 2022 and I am looking forward to the fulfillment of the dream of hosting a television program on healing and restoration.

My encouragement to you dear reader is to know your worth. In order for you to know your worth, you should first know who you are and whose you are. Many of us don't know who we are because all our lives we had to fight: fight molesters, fight haters, fight toxic relationships, fight inner demons, and with all this fighting, we have lost ourselves in the process.

When we know who we are in Christ, we realize that we don't have to fight anymore because we have one fighting for us who has never lost a battle. Also, do not let your past, what others say about you, or even the negative voices in your head determine who you are. Speak words of life over yourself, and remind yourself daily who you are in Christ Jesus. Tell yourself, "I am valuable, I am worth it, and most importantly I am loved."

STEPS TOWARDS INTENTIONAL HEALING

The first thing that I would recommend as you intentionally navigate your way to the other side of grief is prayer, prayer of adoration to God, and prayer of faith.

Use of the word of God: Philippians 4:6-7 (KJV) says, "Do not be anxious about anything but in every situation, by prayer and petition, with thanksgiving, present your requests to God. And the peace of God, which transcends all understanding, will guard your hearts and your minds in Christ Jesus." When you worship and acknowledge God for who He is in your life and pray prayers of praise and faith, God moves on your behalf in miraculous ways causing your anxiety and fears to subside.

Use positive words of affirmation. In Proverbs 18:21 (KJV), the Bible says the power of life and death is in the tongue. It is very important for us to speak words of life over our lives and over the lives of others. Be cognizant of the fact that whatever you say after the words "I am," you will manifest in your life and you will constantly remain in the state of that which you profess. Be deliberate in manifesting positive outcomes by using positive affirmations; for example, you can say, "I am beautiful, I am wonderfully made, and I am blessed."

Lastly, I strive to maintain a positive attitude. It is Charles R. Swindoll who says, "Life is 10% what happens to you and 90% how you react to it." You will find that by cultivating a positive attitude, regardless of how challenging the situation is, changes the atmosphere. When you are able to smile in the midst of your storm, your spirit soars and the difficulties diminish. Through these steps, your scars will become stars.

RESOURCES

Instagram: @ladydsings4u

Facebook: www.facebook.com/ladydministries

Linkedin: www.linkedin.com/in/dawn-lady-d-samuels-lady-d-ministries-859a2a28

CHAPTER 23

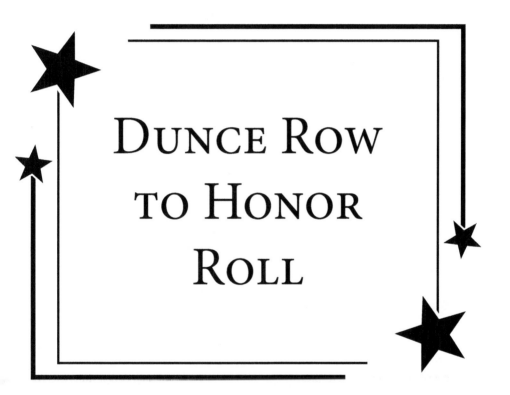

DUNCE ROW TO HONOR ROLL

BY: EVADNE A. MCLILLEY

EVADNE A. MCLILLEY

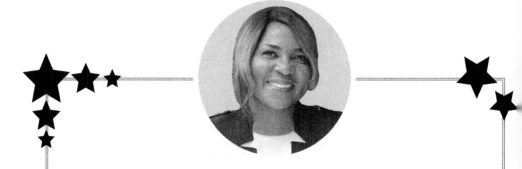

Never stop believing in yourself and your potential to achieve your loftiest dreams, regardless of where or how you started.

A plant-based lifestyle coach, CEO of Ev McLilley Wellness, Inc., Ev McLilley Teas & Herbs and Founder of IMPACT Global Network, Evadne McLilley helps people, especially busy business and executive women, to create a balance between their overactive lifestyle and self-care by teaching them a simple step-by-step, proven method that helps them to eat healthier and reduce stress while finding time for relaxation and self-empowerment.

As Evadne works on building her businesses, she also gives back to society. She created a global outreach movement called IMPACT Global Network to empower young people and encourage people to build better communities and create lasting changes across the world.

Evadne served as president of Junior Chamber International (JCI) – Mandeville Chapter, in Jamaica for three years. She and her team successfully taught young people leadership and project management skills through business and community projects. She was awarded The Mandeville Junior Chamber "10 Outstanding Presidents Award" for Excellence in Leadership at their 25th Anniversary Celebration.

She attended City University of New York, USA and Northern Caribbean University, Jamaica.

Evadne's goal is to impact millions around the world by changing lives and building enterprises and non-profits that will impact generations long after she is gone.

INTENTION

The reader will be inspired by the author's will to not only survive life-threatening childhood illnesses compounded by lack of basic resources, but to later find ways to use those daunting experiences of her childhood to fuel her passion to influence others to be healthy, thrive, and give service to humanity.

DUNCE ROW TO HONOR ROLL

Given the chance to play outside was my standard of a great day as a child. I was restricted to indoors because I was constantly ill. I didn't view my social circumstances as extremely bad at the time because most people in my community had similar economic circumstances. Fortunately, everyone had a roof over their head and food to eat regardless. Life was simple in our farming community, especially for a child.

We learned from early on to make do with what we had and we practiced what mother taught us, "Never go to other people's homes to beg for food or complain that you are hungry." That was a standard house rule so when there was no food, we headed for the "commons" to eat fruits. Sugar cane or ripe bananas from our property were the other options. Gathering and eating fruits was fun, especially during the long summer days. Going out meant going to church next door to beat drums, dance to the negro spiritual songs, participate in concerts, Sunday school, and going on trips to visit other churches if I was well behaved. Not that

I was the type that misbehaved, but I was always a bit on the feisty side.

Summer was my favorite time of year. There was no school, so everyone was home and the kids just played, got dirty, and stopped only to eat. No one supervised us closely really. Strangely, regardless of how hard we fell or how hard someone hit us, none of us suffered a broken bone those days.

When allowed outside, I followed the older kids around, but I had to do what they did or they would not allow me to join them the next time especially if one of my older sisters had anything to do with it. Guess she didn't want Mama up in their business if anything happened to me while being out with them. My mom, Linda, spoiled me rotten. She was a typical mother hen, considering I had several close calls with death. I was not expected to live through those illnesses into adulthood. In fact, my younger sister didn't. We lost her at age four.

Mama, the village unofficial midwife, was very good at keeping the newborns and their mothers alive. She knew a lot about which herbs were good to help cure some illnesses, so I believe she had great lifesaving instincts. I was told those skills were what helped to keep me alive.

According to the Elders and Uncle Egbert, there were many times my mom bawled out from our home perched on top of the hill, "Vadne is dead." My godmother repeatedly shared how the crowd would rush to investigate or confirm my death. Recently while speaking with my sister Vee about this book, she validated the story by sharing that mom kept me alive using her herbal remedies. To this day my favorite uncle Egbert calls me "dead and wake." We have a special bond. I guess every time he looks at me, he marvels that I am still alive. What exactly was the problem is still unclear, but it seems I had asthma and tonsillitis. My tonsils would become so inflamed that they blocked my airway, and it was so critical that I could not breathe. That traumatized Mama. I could not play in the rain. I could not walk anywhere without shoes, and I had to wear a special flannel vest and head covering to "protect me" from getting sick. I can't remember exactly when I stopped getting sick and my protective clothing all fell off but I believe it was shortly after I started school.

With all the ill health drama, Mom didn't allow me to go to school fearing I would get sick and die. I stayed at home until I was seven years old and showed fewer signs of being "sick-sick" before I was allowed to go to school with my siblings. The earlier events created a real-life scar for me because while I was home, no one taught me to read. I had a rocky start at school. Education was not at the top of the agenda, especially for little girls. Sady, my big sister and protector, aged out of that school the year I started. Everything was weird for me because some of the other kids in my class could read and do mental arithmetic but I couldn't.

Life knocked me down when I suffered at the hands of insensitive first and second-grade teachers. They were brutal in their approach and showed no compassion or grace. They didn't try to help me, and they just flogged me with a thick leather strap every time I was not able to read or answer a question correctly. They were rough! I didn't stand a chance with those two. Sometimes if I wasn't beaten with the strap, I got hit with a fist. I was always nervous and scared of being treated so harshly because I was never treated that way at home.

Looking back, I think I survived those two angry ladies because I started to memorize some of the lines from the reading book just by listening to them being read aloud. At some point I could recite "Mr. Joe built a house, Mr. Joe and Miss Tibbs ..." and the rest I would move my mouth like I was reading together in chorus with my classmates.

I never learned to read until I met a calm, patient teacher in the third grade named Mrs. Steel. Not only did I learn to read without her beating me or pressuring me, but I became part of the top nine student group in the class. We used to sit three to a desk, so three desks of us were top of the class of perhaps over forty students. I started to gain confidence and felt like I belonged. I started to run with the bright group and felt comfortable in school and in my skin for the first time. Back then, in order to be in that crowd you had to be bright, be a bully who could fight well, or you had to have some kind of food to feed bullies. I started to fit in because I was bright. I continued to progress academically from there.

Overcoming the hurdle of learning to read eased a lot of pain but the economical struggles didn't change much, so I was not able to continue my education between the ages of fifteen and twenty. I read a lot during those days. I read anything I laid my hands on, sometimes a Harlequin Romance novel per day. I saw the world through books and listening to the radio. I developed a strong sense of who I wanted to be. I made solid friendships with people who cared about my future, usually with people who were more mature, so they pointed me in the right direction. They counseled me from a place of love and respect, so I listened. Following the guidance of my local church Pastor Vincent Peterkin, I applied to West Indies College High School at the age of twenty and was accepted to complete the last three years of high school. I was excited to finally leave my small community to embark on my secondary education journey,

It was not easy paying private high school tuition and rent. I worked on campus for small, unmentionable amounts to help cover tuition. I received assistance from people who acted as angels at the time such as my then Member of Parliament, Neville Lewis, a prominent Montego Bay Attorney who was a solid back-bone type of friend and mentor, and a Manchester-based heavy equipment company that provided a one-year scholarship.

I had a successful academic journey through high school making the honor roll and receiving many awards for outstanding and most outstanding academic performance in different subject areas. Attending the awards function after my first year at high school remains the most meaningful of my entire educational journey. Walking across the stage, I felt accomplished and empowered to do anything and go anywhere using education as a vehicle. I wished my first and second-grade teachers could see me then. As the Jamaican proverb said, "Man no dead, no call dem duppy."

I never really dwelled on why I was so ill when I was a child or why I didn't get the proper medical care that I needed at the time. Removing my tonsils might have solved the problem, but Mom chose not to have them removed and I am now happy she didn't. I also acknowledge that my 1st and 2nd Grade bad experiences inspired me to be an educator many years down the road because I felt strongly that everyone can learn.

I did not question why my first two teachers were so insensitive but rather what personal problems they had that caused them to be so angry. I focused on educating myself, building self-confidence, and learning to thrive regardless of the obstacles I encountered.

Thankfully at age twenty, I threw caution to the wind, listened to people who cared, and made the humbling decision to return to school. I learned to make the quick transition from life as a grown woman to that of a high school girl. Paradoxical as that may sound, it came down to mindset. I was proud of my new life and my surroundings as I settled into life on a beautiful campus. I learned the value of good friendships, tolerance, patience, empathy, forgiveness, self-respect, self-motivation, self-love, self-actualization, and how to inspire others to be helpful.

Arising from my childhood experiences, I have learned these three notable things:

To be persistent, patient and resourceful when teaching a child. If a child does not learn when I am teaching, it is not their failure; it is my failure because I did not figure out a correct way to inspire him or her to learn. Even if that child has cognitive deficiencies or if that child struggles to learn, they can eventually learn, given the right set of circumstances. I took teaching a child to read very personally, as a measure of my success as a classroom teacher. I was passionate about achieving my goals in the classroom and I did.

The power of association can propel me in the right direction and the opposite is also true. From my friends I learned that I could be much more. They were role models I could follow. I grew more self-confident by associating with them. If I didn't have that circle of friends and associates around me to provide positive influence, maybe my choices would have been different. Placing myself in the right environment with the right people has served me well in life from character building to being an upstanding world citizen now influencing others to do the same.

Never give up on myself or my dreams regardless of how impossible they seem. It is not over until it is over. At age 19, I knew I wanted to go back to school but high school was not on my agenda anymore until someone showed me that it was still possible if that's what I wanted. I have proven that the only limit I have is the one I place on myself.

Over the years, I have had different opportunities to teach both adults and children. One priceless opportunity I had was to teach some students in a special education class to catch up academically over a given period. I taught them reading, comprehension, writing, and math skills in one-to-one sessions successfully. I remember placing my hand over some of those kids' hands to help guide them to form letters during handwriting exercises. Thankfully, all got their reading and math levels up, wrote beautifully, and were placed back into their regular classes one to two years later. I was determined to see each of those kids succeed, so I did whatever it took.

Recently, my passion for helping children and adults to read has driven me to create a project to set up a digital reading center in my hometown in Jamaica. I have located a space to accommodate the project and will start implementation in one to two years. I also work to empower young people to become leaders and agents of change in their communities all over. Things are different now for kids in primary school, but I use my influence and platform to encourage others to join me in giving back to schools so more children can escape the scars I suffered and be given the chance to shine like a star from a young age.

Your circumstances do not dictate your final destination. Having setbacks and obstacles in your way may slow you down; they may scar your life too, but they don't have to stop you. Turn your pain into something productive and life-changing. Set out on a mission to ensure that you do what you were placed on this earth to do. Leave no stone unturned. Be bold and take responsibility to lead and change lives. Never stop learning or teaching. You should leave this world empty. Don't leave with all the great ideas in your head. Teach what you know to others. Illuminate the path for them to follow in your footsteps and shine purposely.

The unfortunate circumstances of my early childhood being overshadowed and constricted by illnesses that were treatable have long become distant memories. There is also no excuse to explain away what happened during my first two years of primary school, but I overcame my pain and shame over the years using these three simple steps.

Steps Towards Intentional Healing

The TMO method may work for you if you have had similar experiences and choose to be intentional about your healing as you navigate your scars:

Turn pain and shame into fuel that will drive you to achieve in different areas of your life. Bad things can happen to good people, but how we react to them is what matter the most. Use your pain as fuel to propel you toward greatness. Don't be afraid to use the passion from your pain to drive you towards good.

Make a difference in society. Find meaning and purpose in your life by making a difference in the world. You cannot change the past, but you can help to give someone a better life in many ways. Be a role model to someone. Give back when and where you can.

Own the story and share it to inspire others. By owning your pain, you learn to manage it. Talking about it openly or privately helps you to grow and move on. As you examine your scars, be open to seeing things from all perspectives, not just yours. It will help you to heal. Sometimes, people do bad things because they are hoping those things will lead to the right results. Being open to forgiving someone who wronged you allows you to live your life free of the weight of hate.

Forgiveness is mastery of self. Do yourself a favor: choose to forgive so you can live, not just to merely exist.

Resources

Website: https://evmclilley.com

Instagram: @evmclilleyteas

Facebook: https://www.facebook.com/evmclilley

CHAPTER 24

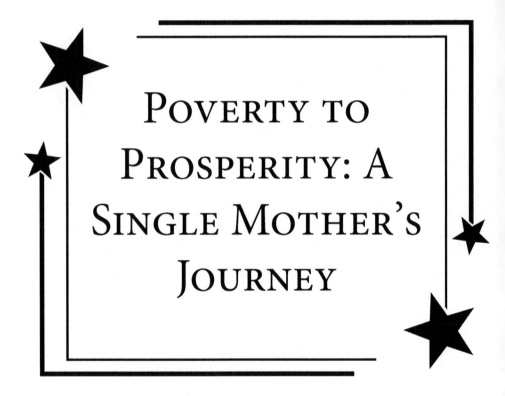

POVERTY TO PROSPERITY: A SINGLE MOTHER'S JOURNEY

BY: JOYCE V. WILLIAMS

Joyce V. Williams

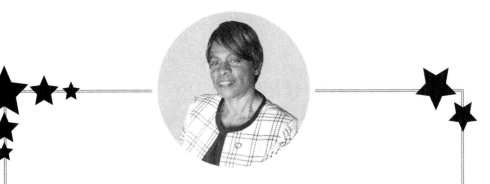

"Motherhood is a God-given gift for a God-driven purpose."
- Joyce Williams

Joyce V. Williams is the proud mother of three children, Keithon, Kenroy, and Roxanne, and grandmother of three grandchildren, Keithon Jr., Shauntae, and Kadian. She values family relationships above self-image and has a passion for children, especially those from low socio-economic backgrounds. Joyce was born and raised in Saint James, Jamaica. She graduated from Northern Caribbean University and served in the ministry of education from 1990-2010 as a nutritionist and home economics educator.

Presently, Joyce is a board member of the Educational Foundation for Children's care (EFCCI), a non-profit organization based in Miami, Florida that provides care for abandoned and indigent children. She is a philanthropist at heart and a great storyteller with international reach. She is the co-founder of the brand Joy-Kissed Creations (JKC), which sells customized apparel, towel sets, and crockery. Joyce also has a passion for learning. She is currently pursuing a degree in Social Work at Miami-Dade College. Her philosophy is "Do all the good you can, by all the means you can, in all the ways you can, to all the people you can, as long as you can." – John Wesley.

INTENTION

Dear reader, if you are a single mother seeking to overcome life's challenges and find your God-given purpose, this story is written for you. My desire is that as you read my story, you will recognize that you were purposefully chosen for motherhood and designed to be the best mother to your children. I encourage you to cherish the love that you have for them. Know that you are not alone and that help is on the way. This story is designed to provide the encouragement you need to propel you toward being successful mothers of valor. My story should inspire you to embrace the unexpected.

POVERTY TO PROSPERITY: A SINGLE MOTHER'S JOURNEY

Life is a journey filled with twists and turns. However, we have the power to control how we perceive our circumstances and create the joy we seek from life even amidst seemingly impossible situations. As I reflect on my life, I recognize that life has not always been good. However, instead of simply allowing life to pull me along its turbulent course, I decided to actively seek out and construct my own world of happiness through my involvement with church, school, and my community. In these moments, life was great.

My first and greatest attempt to find my own joy was to become involved with my local church. What started off as an attempt to feel a part of the church community ended with me having a personal relationship with Jesus Christ and becoming baptized. I could now share my struggles with God and know that He is always listening and guiding me along life's tumultuous path. By taking part and leading in church services, I developed excellent interpersonal and leadership skills that were recognized by many.

School was another avenue for building my happiness. I dreamed of a better life than what I was living, and I recognized that education was a key to success. So, I made it my mission to be fully engaged in learning activities. My achievements gave me a sense of value and pride to see my name listed among the stars. In such moments, life was great.

My exemplary performance at church and school endeared me to the community. I was loved, trusted, and respected by all age groups from young to old. This emboldened me to host a group of children each Sunday afternoon at my house. During these sessions, I discovered and honed my gifts of storytelling, poetry, and teaching. The warm reception from my community improved my self-esteem and allowed me to feel joy despite my poor financial situation.

Books shaped the vision of happiness I wished to create. Whenever I read a book, I was transported to the world in which the characters lived and took part in their lives. I had a vivid picture of the life I wanted to live, my ideal family, and the type of environment in which I wanted my children to be raised.

Altogether, when I decided to take happiness into my own hands, life was great! But inevitably, the unexpected happened several years later.

Growing up as a Christian young lady, I envisioned myself establishing an ideal family life that reflects my religious belief. However, the journey of my life took a different twist. On May 12, 1981, two days after Mother's Day, I celebrated a new life in the form of my first son, Keithon. It was not one of those moments when you would hear congratulations from family or friends. The reality was, I was unmarried, unemployed, and had insufficient resources to take care of myself and my child. However, the very moment that I laid my eyes upon my son's precious face, coupled with his first cry, a love that is indescribable cemented in my heart.

Still, raising a child as a single mother was not easy. There were times when the weight of responsibilities felt unbearable, and I frequently broke down in tears. The self-esteem I carefully built crumbled, and I feared that my life would revert to the way it was when I was younger. Beyond that, I feared that I would bring my son through the same difficulties I faced.

The devastation brought to Jamaica by Hurricane Gilbert compounded my trials. We faced further limitations in securing food, water, and shelter. To make matters worse, my son suffered from regular life-threatening asthma attacks that kept me constantly visiting the hospital. It was unimaginable anguish to watch him suffer but unable to help. My days felt dim and hopeless and I spent many nights on my knees in desperate prayer seeking God's intervention.

Several months later, I went in search of a job, and I noticed a small group of people standing in the courtyard at the Montego-Bay Seventh-Day Adventist Church. I went over to see what it was about and heard the late Pastor L. C. Thomas addressing the group regarding job placement. I quickly booked an appointment with him and told him about my situation, skills, and teaching experience. He sent me to Mrs. Myrie, who invited me to her house to discuss the next steps for employment. During the discussion, she served me a drink and a slice of cake. Instead of eating the cake right away, I discreetly slipped it into my handbag. My action aroused her curiosity and she asked me why I did not eat the cake. I told her I was saving it for my son. Without inquiring further, she packed me a box of food and offered me a part-time position at the end of my visit. I am convinced that it was the Holy Spirit who worked through her to bless me. I still reflect on that day with thanksgiving and joy.

There is one theme that is present throughout my journey from scars to stars. Although there were times that felt dark and hopeless, I always reached out to God for comfort and direction. I also make a conscious effort to reframe my thinking and focus on positive aspects of life, however small.

God gave me the teaching role through Mrs. Myrie, but He knew that I wanted more and that I was hungry for knowledge. By faith, I enrolled at Northern Caribbean University because I had no money to pay for my tuition. God provided for me through the school's work-study program; I was offered a full-time position as a cook in the school cafeteria. I was able to attend classes and studied in the evenings and at nights. During those periods, my son was loved and cared for by a close relative. The years I spent at school were far from easy, but I took courage from Jeremiah 29:11 (NIV), "For I know the plans I have for you, plans to prosper you and not to harm you, plans to give you hope and a future." Within the trials of working and studying, I met life-long friends and recommitted my life to God. After three successful years, my son was able to watch me proudly stride across the graduation stage with an Associate degree in home economics and food preparation. With this degree, and other educational achievements, I served the ministry of education for 20 years as a high-school instructor. During this time, I got married and was blessed with two other children: Kenroy and Roxanne.

Again, God saw my desire for a better future for myself and my family. In His omniscience, He allowed my mother to traverse and overcome the rugged path of migrating to the U.S.A. so that she could be the gateway through which my family and I crossed in 2010. Indeed, it is through my mother's vision and determination to fight for the betterment of her family that her children and grandchildren are in the U.S.A. today.

My arrival in the U.S.A. gave me the opportunity to achieve most of my long-term goals. I learned to drive, got a good paying job, bought a car and a house, and am now pursuing a Bachelor's degree in social work. With my children grown and successful in their own right, I have taken up learning a new language and playing the keyboard. I also volunteer for a non-profit organization that provides help for children that are less fortunate. As Ken Robinson once said, "What you do for yourself dies with you when you leave this world; what you do for others lives on forever."

My journey has been a rocky one, but I am grateful for the scars for they tell my story. Having my first child out of wedlock seemed like a loss of self and integrity. I sank deeply into despair and grieved for the "me" I imagined as a child as one would grieve the loss of a close family member. Now that I have been through the process of grieving, healing, and restoration, I can now embrace grieving as a normal response to any pain and loss. To all who are in their moment of grieving, know that there is healing on the other side.

As a single mother going through the valley of my own experiences, I thought there was no way out of my despair. The fear and anxiety I felt during this time were almost crippling. But, I found hope in the small things in life. Sunny days, blue skies, calm winds, and laughter lifted my spirit and gave me the motivation to move forward one step at a time. Caring for my son, which was a source of hardship, became my delight when I decided to be thankful for all that I had. My son was alive and well, always had food to eat, and was properly clothed despite my struggles.

This gave me further joy and strength. Moreover, I am grateful for my family and friends who were my constant cornerstones of support in my time of need. Enduring the challenges I faced as a single mother taught me to embrace the unexpected. Furthermore, I discovered skills, such as multitasking, collaboration, and negotiating, that I didn't know I had. I am grateful for the courage and resilience that I have gained. Now I know that instead of worrying when things go awry, I will express gratitude and show my children unconditional love. The unexpected will happen, but when you love through it, brighter days will be ahead.

When I reminisce about my life's journey as a single mother, I smile with a sense of gratitude. My self-esteem took a huge hit when I had my first son, but God was with me every step of the way. I learned that I am still loved and a treasured child of God. I redeveloped my self-esteem and self-respect and grew in my sense of responsibility and self-confidence. I am now more loving, caring, and forgiving. I have the fortified courage to stand up to the task of motherhood with pride and integrity. I have admired the progress of my children, and how they grew from uncertainty to gratitude and from pain to possibility. I felt encouraged that the God who started a good work will carry it to completion. Indeed, God has given me a roadmap to succeed. Sometimes I get distracted on the journey, but I learned how to maneuver in love. Rumi quotes, "Love is a mirror. In it you see nothing except your reflection."

Despite the challenges in my life, I found ways to be grateful and positive avenues through which to restore my passion and purpose in life. I spent quality time in meditation during which I focused on ways to balance my life and the well-being of others. I formed and maintained valued friendships with people who helped me to see the good in me and were honest enough to show me my weakness. Their influence has informed my goal of crafting a mentorship program for young women facing financial challenges in their pursuit of education to attain a profitable way of self-improvement.

I am empowered to help single mothers discover and develop their God given talents and be able to look beyond the temporary problems they are encountering. I assist single mothers by providing useful information on how to maintain good health, both physically and mentally and ways to access emergency care. I am also a board member of a non-profit organization that provides food, shelter, and clothing for abandoned and indigent children in the Caribbean. Seeing these initiatives change the lives of single mothers and children is as much a blessing to me as it is to those they benefit.

You may have become a single mother through the loss of a spouse, financial challenges, ignorance, looking for love in the wrong place, or simply the results of a dysfunctional home. Whatever your situation, there is hope. You are much more than what society labels you. You are a woman with dignity, integrity and pride. Keep chasing your dreams; it is never too late to go back to school, learn a new language, or learn a skill. There is nothing that God cannot do in your lives. Remember, there is power in prayer. May the words penned by Don Moen be your consolation, "God will make a way where there seems to be no way. He works in ways we cannot see. He will be my guide, hold me closely to His side, with love and strength for each new day."

STEPS TOWARDS INTENTIONAL HEALING

Three action steps toward intentional healing as you navigate from scars to stars are:

Step 1: Value Yourself. As single mothers, we may feel that we must discard ourselves for our children. However, in the same way that the airplane safety instructions say to put on your own mask before helping to put on a mask on the child, we need to take care of ourselves mentally and physically to be able to take care of others. Success comes only when we give our best to fulfill our needs and be of service to others.

Step 2: Say Yes to Progress, No to Regrets. Someone once said, "When you heal the memories from your past, you start to see the present differently." Do not allow the past to control your future. Your pregnancy may be unplanned, or conceived out of wedlock, but remember, every child is God's heritage and should be treated as such. They are a part of your life, specially designed by the Almighty.

Step 3: Think like a Winner. Life's journey is like a race. For you to be successful, you must be prepared to leave the starting line. But before you take off, you'll face the countdown: "On your mark" – pray for spiritual guidance; "Get set" – remember your passion; "Go" – chase towards your goals. Never give up; you are a winner!

RESOURCES

Facebook: @journeytojoyce

CHAPTER 25

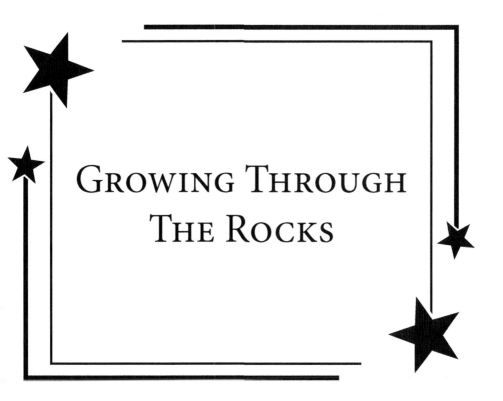

GROWING THROUGH THE ROCKS

BY: **DR. PATRICE WRIGHT**

DR. PATRICE WRIGHT

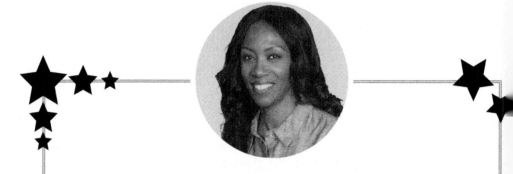

"Overcoming challenges prepares one to overcome greater challenges which inspire the wise." - Patrice Wright

Dr. Patrice Wright has been an educator for over 30 years and has taught kindergarten through college level students. She has served primarily as a high school English teacher. As an educator, her goal is to transform lives so that individuals will contribute in a positive way to society and have heaven as their goal. She is a mother of two adult married children and a grandmother of six. She obtained a PhD degree in leadership at Andrews University and presently teaches college students.

INTENTION

Behind every dark cloud is a silver lining. In addition to this reality, the author intends for readers to understand that rewards are derived from one's best efforts. Brought to view is appreciation is not always experienced while one is accomplishing his or her task, but often experienced at the end of it. The value of stick-to-itiveness is emphasized. Characteristics such as being willing to handle unwelcome situations effectively are unfolded. This chapter reveals that life's experiences are opportunities for developing positive attributes. It is hoped that the pages' contents will be a source of encouragement.

GROWING THROUGH THE ROCKS

Dressed in my gray skirt suit and orange top, I stepped out the front door with my handbag and large rolling computer case filled with books and other teacher resource materials including my laptop. I locked my front door, stepped in my black Toyota Camry and was off to work at 7:00 A.M. I arrived at my workplace at 7:35 A.M. This was a routine occurrence for approximately 20 years. Teaching high school students who entered my class with a blank look and, at times unruly behavior, was a joyful experience. For I had the opportunity to build a relationship and pour knowledge in approximately 150 students daily and guide them in being respectful to their peers, administrators, teachers, parents, and me.

I still remember the student who, during the first week of class, pretended he was a flying airplane. How disturbing this ninth grader was! Other teachers constantly complained about him. I immediately involved him in just about every activity I could think of from erasing the chalkboard, answering questions, and eliciting classroom discipline protocol ideas from him. By the second week, he was one of my best-behaved students. Additionally, as a dean of discipline, I had the autonomy to curb the behavior of students.

At the beginning of each term, I shared my goals with the class. I informed students that I expected the highest levels of development from them and assured them that they could meet these expectations. I aligned my objectives, instructional strategies, and assessments to provide a comprehensive picture of what was expected of students. I usually spent the first day of class reviewing the syllabus with students and providing them with an opportunity to indicate ways in which it could better satisfy their needs. I believed in the importance of an integrated education and modeled this belief by incorporating in my lessons literature from various disciplines.

I always created a comfortable classroom climate. This was achieved by expressing sensitivity to diverse learners as I addressed their needs and celebrated the culture of students in several ways. I employed various teaching approaches to promote student engagement in learning such as direct instruction, cooperative learning, jigsaw strategy, Socratic seminars, and vocabulary acquisition. I also utilized technology to support instruction. I believe that making learning fun, tangible, and memorable creates an environment for peak learning. I enjoyed teaching. Administrators, teachers, students, and parents appreciated me.

I encountered the custodian in the hallway who told me that my high school and others in the area would close. As faculty, we were encouraged to do all in our power to improve student success rates in the regents and local examinations. At times, I arrived at work at 7:35 A.M. and left at 9:00 P.M. I felt the sacrifice was worth every ounce of my effort in order that our dear school would be kept afloat. There were endless evaluations from the state and city education department. In the end, our school closed. I was devastated. The school I called home no longer belonged to me.

To add fuel to fire, I was offered a permanent teaching position two years prior to our school's closing but was not released from my school to accept this much sought-after position. I suspect the principal saw the need to have an effective English teacher as part of the faculty. I was devastated.

The financial perks of teaching after school, covering additional classes, and my involvement in various afterschool programs ended. These were a source of income for my children who attended college. We would not meet many of our administrators, colleagues, and students again. We were a group of mourners. Most of us applied to be permanently placed in a school within this education system but for the most part, our requests were not honored. There were unspoken reasons for these very many negative responses.

Soon we learned we were classified as ATRs (Absent Teacher Reserve) who would be sent from school to school serving in a similar way a substitute teacher does. Fear stems from the unknown, and this emotion was revealed by our questions. Would we be terminated? How would we sustain ourselves? How would our children in college be adequately provided for? How would our mortgages be paid? Would we be able to retire with benefits from the system? The questions were endless and there were no answers in sight.

Conversations among ATRs were expressed in whispers, phone calls, irate voices, uncouth language, and threats of various kinds such as lawsuits, but all seem to have been of no effect. I learnt from one of these interactions with my fellow colleagues that a retired administrator was offered a job to evaluate ATRs as unsatisfactory to give credence for their termination. My heart pounded. Many left the teaching profession.

I stayed. I had faith that God, who provided me with this teaching position, would not leave me without bread. I would persevere and depend on Him. I now had no fear. Initially, we ATRs were sent to various schools. At first we experienced weekly rotations, then monthly, then yearly and at times, we were placed in schools, as needed. We could not predict the school where we would be placed. I felt unfairly punished but decided to do my best. I thought, "I am God's child and He wants me to reflect His character." Hence, as I taught each class, I did my best. I treated my students as if I were their assigned teacher. I now began experiencing the joy of teaching once again.

Regardless of the schools I was assigned, I built relationships with students, incorporated life skills in my teaching, and soon began to feel appreciated by the administration, faculty, staff, students, and parents. Upon arrival at one of the schools, the assistant principal of English shouted, "Welcome Ms. Wright. We are so happy to have you back." I felt celebrated. On departure, one of the administrator's voiced, "We will miss you." I was overjoyed.

September came around again, and I anxiously awaited my new high school assignment. I opened the familiar letter, and to my chagrin it read, "You are assigned to _____ Elementary School." "Elementary school!" I cried. "How dare they?" I stopped in my tracks. Immediately, I turned to God, bowing my head and whispered, "Your will be done."

I worked untiringly seeking to understand methods, learning styles, and interests of these elementary students, for I was in unfamiliar territory. All seemed a challenge. It felt more comfortable to teach high school students physics compared to teaching these little ones. However, I took time to prepare lessons for classes. In cases where the lessons were inadequate, I filled the gap.

One day, the principal called me to her office requesting that I teach grade four for three months while the classroom teacher went on maternity leave. I hesitantly accepted. I knew I had to keep a stiff upper lip.

Math, the subject I dreaded, strangely became my favorite subject to teach. The other grade four teachers were supportive. The inordinate hours I invested in preparation made teaching effective. In addition to the classroom resources I possessed, I frequently sought guidance and ensured that students were orderly and productive.

Surprisingly, I received a letter from a parent, Mrs. Irene Raevsky, expressing her gratitude to me for teaching her daughter. I was encouraged. A few years passed, and my yearly rotation from school to school continued.

As I sat at the dining room table eating my sweet and sour tofu, rice and peas, tossed salad and steamed string beans, my mind was diverted by the ringing phone. "Hello!" On the other side of the phone, I heard a happy, crying, and breathless voice. "We were trying to find you. My daughter is in tears right now. To no avail, she spent days trying to find your telephone number. I assisted her. I am so happy we found you." Irene Raevsky continued to tell me that I inspired her daughter, Kristina, who I taught in fourth grade, to write a book. Mrs. Raevsky arranged that I join the family at brunch. There I received an autographed copy of Fly Me to the Moon and Other Stories. I beamed as I saw my name in the acknowledgment section. Presently, Kristina is a junior high student and has completed her second book.

The fruits of my labor had come to fruition.

Have you ever felt that at any time your world may cave in? Those thoughts permeated my mind when my school was closed and my future seemed unpredictable. Regardless of what was transpiring in the school system, I decided not to quit, to do my best, and to depend on God, the source of my strength. My experience demonstrated that the way life's nightmares are addressed leads to success, mediocrity, or failure. What if I had quit? My retirement benefits would have been adversely affected. The income to support my children's college education would be uncertain. My day-to-day source of sustenance may be in the balance, and today I would not have been experiencing the blessings of my resolve.

Why me was a question that resounded frequently in my head. I felt like a homeless person when my school closed and I was constantly sent to various high schools, as well as an elementary school. I felt as if I had lost my dear school family and the respect I gained as a teacher.

Despite the discomfort from the experience, I am grateful to have been provided the opportunity to serve in various schools. The opportunity offered invaluable knowledge of how administrators, teachers, and students functioned effectively or ineffectively. Personally, as an educator, I was nurtured.

I am also appreciative of the relationships I formed with teachers and administrators. The rich resources gleaned from them continues to support my ability to teach in new and innovative ways. Students and parents also enriched my journey preparing me to be better equipped to relate to various cultures. Instead of asking why me, I now ask, why not me? To upset the apple cart can also be a good idea.

Being displaced from the school I served for approximately 20 years was painful. This experience generated invaluable life lessons such as not quitting, doing my best, and accentuating the positive. I recall that when the school I called my own closed, several teachers and administrators who worked there left their jobs. They chose not to endure the seeming hardship of being rotated from school to school.

The benefits of not quitting are at times monetary. Additionally, stick-to-itiveness develops character. For in dealing with everyday problems and situations, it is important to see these to completion. This elicits appreciation by you and others, for then the value of work is on full display. As we interact and work with individuals, it is paramount to offer encouragement, and to notify them of their growth and strengths. This important aspect of character development was evidenced when I told Kristina, my fourth-grade student, that she would be an outstanding writer. Today, as a six grader, she has written two books. Character traits such as not quitting, doing our best, and accentuating the positives are vital character development elements for successfully surmounting and navigating over life's hurdles and around life's darts.

In retrospect, I shivered at being displaced from the school I called my own. Each classroom, hallway, office, and gym created feelings of nostalgia. On my bookshelf at home sits books such as Hamlet, Their Eyes Were Watching God, and The Color of Water. These elicit similar emotions. By contrast, I am comforted that the nightmare is now behind me. This turning point emanated from putting my trust in God. His leadership and guidance steered me in a path where I see challenges as an obstacle that I must overcome, for such experiences are a preparation to successfully deal with greater challenges. People are inspired by the successes of others. Hence, I refuse to quit and seek to inspire and encourage others.

Reflecting on my challenges brings the awareness that the frequent school rotations I endured provided ample time that contributed to my progress in the PhD program. It also afforded an abundance of knowledge of how other schools functioned.

Today, I have completed my PhD program, and my various experiences within numerous schools have provided an invaluable educational resource. Now I am better equipped as an educator to serve. God is my source of empowerment. All glory goes to Him.

The words of one of my favorite songs, "Be not dismayed whate'er betide, God will take care of you," encapsulates the mindset that underlies overcoming challenges. These words serve as an antidote to being distraught, crestfallen, and believing that no one seems to listen nor care. For the vicissitudes of life can be besetting.

When life deals you hard punches, press on. When there seems no way out, do not despair. God will never leave you nor forsake you. His hands are outstretched, just waiting for you to reach out to Him. Nightmares experienced in careers, relationships, death, sickness, finances, depression, and inability to have freedom of choice can be overcome. Lay your burdens at Jesus' feet and embrace His promise that He will take care of you. Look to the Savior. Surrender your life totally to Him. My scars became directional stars, and so can yours.

STEPS TOWARDS INTENTIONAL HEALING

As you seek to heal intentionally and navigate your scars, here are three proven steps:

Remember God is faithful. Do not give up even when the road is difficult to navigate. Keep going. This is part of your character-building journey. At the end of each segment of your journey, you will be stronger and have learnt several life lessons. Hence, you will be prepared to effectively navigate more difficult hurdles.

Tackle your task meticulously. Do your best. This encapsulates being there for others in the best way possible. This is an effective way of taking the focus off you, hence minimizing your challenges, pain, suffering, grief, and burdens. As you encourage others and their characters grow, the joy you receive will have a healing effect on your life.

Blessings come from God. He provides the strength and the power needed for us to deal with every situation. All our abilities come from him. We are encouraged by good experiences and molded by the bad ones. These foster spiritual growth and transform us to reflect God's image. Going through the furnace with God makes us stronger and finer. Thus we are healed, we are overcomers, and we are conquerors.

RESOURCES

Linktree: https://linktr.ee/pdou9999

Facebook: patrice.douglas.56.

CHAPTER 26

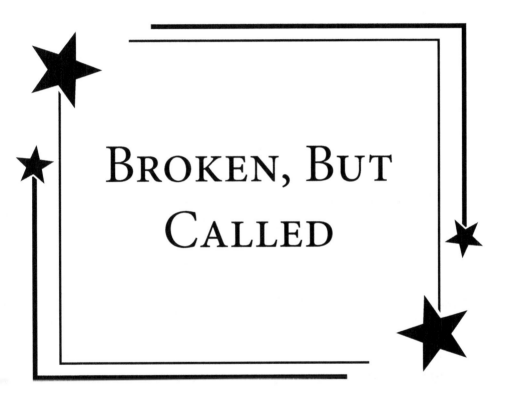

BROKEN, BUT CALLED

BY: **CLAUDIA V. FRANCIS**

CLAUDIA V. FRANCIS

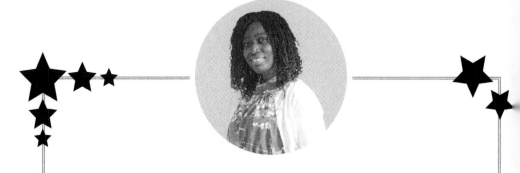

"Your fiery furnaces are refining you for greatness while your obstacles are opportunities for your blessings."
- Claudia V. Francis

Chaplain Claudia V. Francis is a board-certified chaplain in the United Kingdom and United States of America. She currently serves as Senior Chaplain of Mental Health and Learning Disability at the Royal Cornhill Hospital, Aberdeen Scotland. She has amassed a wealth of experience in palliative care, trauma, mental health, and pediatric chaplaincy.

Chaplain Francis has journeyed in the trenches with Veterans, traversed the challenges of inner-city Detroit, journeyed through the unknown, expanded her wings, numbed from her encounters, faced her fears, as God reauthored her story, redirected her focus, redefined her purpose, and revealed the power of presence. Warmed by the charms, hearts, smiles, relentless fight, and compelling faith of her patients, God ignited her passion for hospital chaplaincy.

Chaplain Claudia is a fellow of the Association of Chartered Certified Accountants, with over 20 years' experience in accounting and auditing. She has a passion for preaching and is an international speaker and presenter. She has written several drafts of her life encounters and looks forward to sharing with you her journey from the deskside to the bedside. God has used her mosaic heritage and her past profession as tools in her kits as He uses brokenness to heal brokenness.

INTENTION

My hope is that as you journey through my encounter, you will discover that irrespective of where you are, and the choices that you have made, that God can work even in the seemingly difficult situations in your life for the greater good. You will recognize you are never too far that God cannot rescue you, redirect you, and give you a new mandate. You will appreciate that God has equipped you for ministry, will use you the greatest when you are at your lowest, and use your brokenness as connector points and opportunities of healing for others.

BROKEN, BUT CALLED

It was like a light bulb went off in my head. Suddenly, somewhere between going to bed and waking up, my purpose was transformed from a life of trial and error, twists, and turns. My young mind grappled as I oscillated between professions that captivated my attention. My love and passion to become an astronaut, pilot, lawyer, and everything legal, including a judge, was now in the periphery as God planted His dreams in my mind that night. I recognized then that He had a different plan for my life, and I was sold on it. My passion for the things of God grew immensely. I started to hunger and thirst for Him in new and interesting ways. My peers and family thought I was weird and unambitious as I slowly lost interest in everything except evangelism, outreach, preaching, and finding ways to make money.

I spent the ensuing years knowing that I was called and was confident about it. I was alienated but my naturally reserved nature meant that I was not the least disturbed by this alienation. Despite the challenge of being a woman and the fact that many thought this meant God could not use me, I was on top of the world. If I were good enough to do anything else called ministry, I was just as good to be a pastor, and that was enough to prod me along. I was in the church long enough to know that it would be a struggle, but I was undeterred. So determined was I that I started The First Singles Club to motivate singles to use their talent in His service. Many thought we were simply seeking spouses, so I joked about starting the first Seventh-day Adventist convent. It was fun! I had several oppositions to my plans and ideas for ministry as the norm was every girl wanted to get married. The prevailing opinion was that I was unrealistic and unambitious. I decided that I did not want to spend my life trying to fit in with the churches' mold and blends, so I decided to be a missionary.

Euphoria is short-lived in this life. One day I felt strange pains and shortness of breath as I lay in my dorm room. Back then I did not realize it, but now I know. I had been experiencing a day of death aura as I projected my mother's last moments of life. Three months later, my grief was compounded by the death of my paternal grandfather who lived in the same household. I was estranged from my "friends" and went into a reclusive mode. Now disenfranchised and encountering several health challenges, I was tossed to and fro on the tide of all that was happening in my life and my disconnect with others. While still coming to terms with my loss, I emigrated to the United Kingdom.

God reaffirmed my calling, but my distraction by life's happenings impacted me. I was wading in uncharted territories separated from the norms, religious community, friends, and family. Life then could be summed up in the words of Considering Lily's song, "My life was like a jigsaw with missing pieces, square pegs, and round holes, like trying to climb a ladder but always slipping, high jump, short pole..." There was never a dull moment. I encountered many perils, isolated in church, work, and even my friendship circle. That was the price for being different – racially, ethnically, spiritually, and characteristically. It was continuous and each blessing came with deeper challenges, institutional discrimination, abuse, displacement, statelessness, immigration abuse, hospitalization, financial losses, barrenness, and broken-heartedness.

The continuity of my struggles was confusing; God had gone silent for too long. I could not see His plan and I was struggling and tired of others trying to squeeze me into their own mold. One day, I met a colleague who was trying to redirect my ministry. He was drowning in his own ministry, but I failed to realize this until it was too late as I was busy wondering about his interest in my ministry. I resisted the Holy Spirit's urge to call him that morning only to later learn of his suicide. I could not undo the past, so I surrendered. Seminary was but a segment of the journey. After a near-death experience and Clinical Pastoral Education dramas, I returned to audit and accounting, but God ensured He got my attention.

God's relentless pursuit of me became evident after I was smoked out ten times, hospitalized for four days, and benched from traveling for work. Exhaustion coupled with emotional unavailability, I struggled to identify one Bible character with whom I could associate. Job did not resonate with me as I never got my plenty, just more troubles than before. I had volumes of journals, fasted, and prayed, pouring out my heart to God. My pillows were stained from the nightly tears. I recognized that the more I told God I had enough, the more my troubles magnified. Physically, emotionally, and spiritually tired after my Friday night worship, I cried out to the Lord, prostrated, and presented my prayer request like King Hezekiah. I pleaded with the Lord for 6 months of Jubilee for my years of continuous problems. Rising from my knees, I found myself singing words from Laura Story's song "Blessing," "What if your blessings come through raindrops? What if your healing comes through tears? What if a thousand sleepless nights are what it takes to know You're near? And what if trials of this life are Your mercies in disguise?..." I realized as I journeyed to start my Clinical Pastoral Education that God was telling me the journey would be difficult.

After deep introspection, I acknowledged that I was vacillating in the way I dealt with my problem. I needed to choose either to toughen up like an egg in boiling water or soften like a carrot under the pressure of heat. I decided I needed to be a coffee bean, to change my circumstances when pressured by heat. I needed to focus on the size of my God and not the size of my problems. I started to change the way I prayed, spending quality time in His presence, giving thanks daily as often as I could. "Tis So Sweet To Trust in Jesus" was my daily song, and the only words that made sense were, "Oh for grace to trust Him more." I was learning to hold on to faith, traversing the labyrinth, many redirections, new paths, unlearning and learning, wrestling with God while learning to grow and bloom in pain. I stopped asking God to remove the problems and challenging people. Instead, I asked for Him to grant me strength and for Him to carry me through as He had promised. The words of the Psalms were like meat unto my soul as I sought to impregnate my mind with praise.

Although nothing in my life had changed, with the shift in my focus, God anointed my eyes to start to see things through His lenses. I was more intentional in my prayer for the Holy Spirit to reveal the things that needed changing and to break generational curses so that it would stop with me. I learned to trust what I know about God. He never removed my problems. The struggles I faced with remuneration, licensing, and quality of treatment persisted, but God transformed me. He used my struggles as character refinement tools. God affirmed me through my patients, even when I did not feel good enough. He provided healing when the doctors pronounced doom. Divine grace and favor permeated my life as He brought me through and shut the mouth of the lions. I gave God full permission to ignore my cries and pleads and to grant only what was according to His will, showered with grace and favor. His sharpening tools are now connector points that help me to minister to my patients. My challenges, setbacks, and experiences were vehicles of transport for my next blessings.

I was fixated on my nosocomephobia, necrophobia, hemophobia, and germaphobia. Why would God allow me to lose the job that was supposed to pay my way and compound that problem when I got sick with an undiagnosable, untreatable disease? But God has orchestrated every minute of my experience and was rerouting my pathway. He was using my perceived deficiencies to prepare me for the work He was about to launch me into as He rewired my mental circuitry and detoxed my thoughts. Through prayer, praise, journaling, Bible reading, and forgiveness, I eliminated my negative self-talk of "I don'ts" and "I cant's." Replacing them with "I can do this" and "this too shall pass," I mastered true dependence on God and purpose and embraced His grace. My clinical pastoral education, the hospitals I worked in, and patients encountered were building up the resources that I could pull from. My analytic skills, assiduousness, and vigilance with finding the unknown were skills that enhanced my chaplaincy. Problems, pain and setbacks were reauthored as challenges, mercies, and blessings in disguise. God used every detail of my life as connector points that helped me to meet the diverse needs of the patients that I minister to daily.

Intentional Healing: From Scars to Stars

Toxicity is not just about the relationships that we have but also the negative thoughts that we have allowed ourselves to believe as factual. As I surrendered to the work that God was doing in my life, I was able to flourish. My focus encountered a 180° shift as I started to seek ways of improving the quality of life of others who were in adverse circumstances and championed the cause of the downtrodden. I had weathered the storms of affliction and abuse so others needed to catch a vision of the fact that they could do the same. Emerging stronger after my experience, I seek to encourage others to be strong and assist persons in their struggles. A combined effort is always better than going the journey alone. My experience enabled me to be more compassionate and empathetic as I decided to become an agent of change for others. Actively listening, I am able to affirm, mentor, guide, and encourage others. God's promises are true; with courage, I have embraced my calling. I no longer suffer in silence, and I encourage others to be better versions of themselves and to actualize their potential.

Intentionally blooming in the murky waters of pain like the lily does in a stagnant pond was a decision I made. As I daily surrendered to God and invited the Holy Spirit to take control, I found that the scars of my past were no longer the central focus of my life. An intensified prayer life buffered my life at home, walking the corridors and even when with patients. I am humbled how God ministered to me through my patients. My journey through and subsequent healing amidst pain helps me to minister to the needs of patients who face their struggles with life's circumstances. The hope that I have embraced helps me to seek to lead them to embrace hope as well and catch a glimpse of light in their darkness. I take mental health breaks when life becomes toxic, regroup, set boundaries, and exercise self-care. Additionally, I developed rituals to detach work from home; one of the greatest helps was this new confidence of owning my pastoral identity. This enables me to not just meet patients where they are but to guide them on a path of greater self-awareness and embracing their personal giftedness and personhood.

DeMarcus Cousins wrote, "God gives his hardest battles to his strongest soldiers." Jacob the supplanter contended with God and obtained favor. Joseph went from pit to prison to palace but never lost sight of his dreams and the God who gave it to him and granted him favor. Jabez was destined to a life of pain but prayed to God to rewrite his story and never let him bring pain, to bless him and broaden his territory.

No one thought David had potential, but God chose him as His king. He waited a possible 20 years gaining firsthand experience through difficulty for the crown. Jeremiah was selected for a life of singleness and preaching doom and gloom. Paul was beaten with rods, shipwrecked three times, pelted with stones, and jailed, but he stayed the course. Like these men and women of faith, be encouraged and stay the course because God has chosen you.

Steps Towards Intentional Healing

There are several steps toward being intentional about your healing; however, I would like to share three of them with you.

When God calls, know His voice, and recognize that some dreams are only for your ears. Spiritual things are spiritually discerned. There are always good, intentional individuals who "know" what is best and will veer you away from God's plans. Don't disqualify your call. Your past is your past and you can make a fresh start. Just say yes to God's call. He will reauthor your story and redirect your purpose.

Trust the process. Your call to ministry is not dependent on worldly connectedness. Avoid comparing your success with man's criteria. Flowers differ in their cultivation process; however, they all bloom with radiance. So, be confident that if God calls you, He has already fixed you, and will equip you for the call. He has faith in you. Keep your eyes on Him and not on the challenges. Seek Him earnestly, be audacious knowing that anywhere you go with Jesus is safe. Embrace the challenges and continuity; your call is not defined by your struggles. Your fiery furnaces are refining you for greatness while your obstacles are opportunities for your blessings. He who starts the work for you is faithful to complete it.

Pursue righteousness and put God first and everything will fall into place. Don't be afraid to put God to the test; give Him back His words and promises, never trust in your feelings, fast, pray, and praise. It can be difficult to seek God when life becomes broken, but be transparent about your feelings. Now stand still and watch God fight for you, as He lifts you from the ashes, and like an Iris, He elevates you out of the mire and lets you bloom where you are planted.

Resources

LinkedIn: c-f-1915ba231

YouTube: www.youtube.com/channel/UCoRQKbTAnN-joZ9fp7NI5sw

Instagram: Baal.peratsiym22

CHAPTER 27

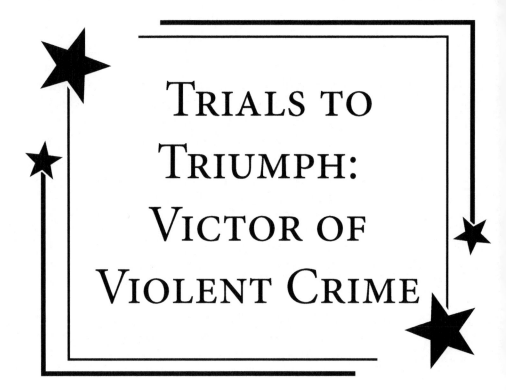

TRIALS TO TRIUMPH: VICTOR OF VIOLENT CRIME

BY: ROY PUSEY

ROY PUSEY

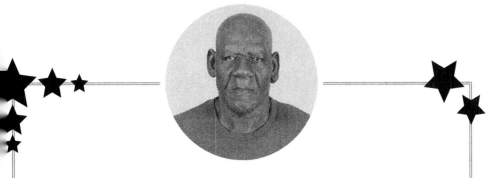

Don't be crippled by the impact of violence. You can walk away, and you don't always have to fight back. It feels great to forgive those who have done you wrong. - Roy Pusey
Blessed is the man that walketh not in the counsel of the ungodly, nor standeth in the way of sinners. - Psalm 1:1 (KJV)

Mr. Roy Pusey hails from the parish of Clarendon in the community of York Town. He is a dedicated father and husband. He has been married for twenty six years and fathered five children, three sons and two daughters. Though not confined to any specific occupation, Mr. Pusey worked as a heavy equipment operator for several years. He also worked odd jobs to boost the family income. In the truest sense of the word, Mr. Pusey is a family man, as he often boasts of helping with the household chores and the love he has for his children. He describes himself as a hard-working individual who is always on the move. His wife describes him as a good father, always going the extra mile to make his family happy. Mr. Pusey loves to farm and he plants anything, from a pea to a mango tree. He has a deep love for aesthetics which is manifested in the beautiful flowers and well kept manicured lawn at his home. When he is not practicing his horticultural skills, he enjoys watching a good Western or cowboy movie.

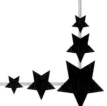

INTENTION

My purpose is to share my story outside of the confines of my community. I want people across the world to know my story and to let them know that they should not allow themselves to be crippled by the impact of violence. It is my hope that my story will bring hope to persons who have been impacted by violence one way or the other.

TRIALS TO TRIUMPH: VICTOR OF VIOLENT CRIME

My family consisted of my wife, Kat, three sons (Tas, Carr, and Rom), and two daughters (Van and Ran). We live in Bullard Content, York Town, Clarendon. Our family had limited resources, but we shared a loving relationship. To us, life was great. We were satisfied with what we had. We were happy just doing our best. In 2006, because of her daughter's health concerns, my wife Kat grabbed the opportunity to go visit and be with our daughter in Canada. While she was there, I received a little more financial assistance. I was always the only one working and taking care of the family. My children and I had some great times even though I was working very hard to provide for and nurture them, having been left with the motherly role while still trying to be a great father with Kat not around. Our four kids were going to school and it was very hard on me financially. When I left work in the evening, I would have to take care of the domestic side of the home. In spite of all of these demands, I was still enjoying a great life with my children. They were jovial and very funny at times. I remember when life was just great!

INTENTIONAL HEALING: FROM SCARS TO STARS

On July 8, 2011, I was at a grave digging next door to our house to offer neighborly assistance and support. I was there for about 15 minutes when tragedy struck. Gunmen invaded and shot up the graveside. I was feared dead with ten gunshot wounds in my leg and foot. I was rushed to the May Pen Hospital where I was admitted for two days and was later transferred to the Mandeville Regional Hospital for further treatment. This was devastating for the entire family. We couldn't control our grief because I was the sole breadwinner for the family and my wife was still away, but God was in the midst.

During this difficult period, my eldest son would travel to the Mandeville Hospital to take care of me. At home, my eldest daughter had to be playing the role of mother for her other two siblings. It was very challenging but as a family, we were fighting and determined to move forward, from scars to stars. During this time, I was still in the hospital doing test after test, surgery after surgery, and it was overwhelming. It felt more like being sunken in a dark dungeon with a tiny glimpse of hope. This one random act of violence threw my family into a tailspin of devastating events. On February 13, 2013, my wife returned home to Jamaica. By then, I was out of the hospital, but I couldn't walk. She immediately released Vanessa and fell back into her motherly role. The financial obligations were insurmountable. My children's education was at stake. By faith, Van applied to a university and was successful. She started her journey to success.

Rom, my 3rd son, was out of school and unemployed. My youngest daughter was also unemployed. Romario aspired to go to university. However, despite my fears and objections, he started working on a construction site in the nearby community to supplement the family's income. In 2021, violence struck my family again. Our eldest son, a father of four, was fatally shot. We were devastated. Still challenged with my ordeal, my wife spiraled into a state of shock and confusion, not knowing where to turn. Life really knocked us down hard!

While we were still down, we were receiving support from family, friends, and the wider community. I was really grateful. It's been 11 years on and I am just learning to walk again. To say that life was difficult after my incident and later on the brutal killing of our son is mild. It was like a windstorm in my head. My wife was struck hardest as she was left to carry the burden of the family. The children bore their pain in different ways. Seeing how they hurt, I believe no one should have to live through such pain inflicted by violence.

With a strong sense of loss, I had to decide to take action toward healing my emotional scars like I did the physical wounds to my legs. While still living in the crime-prone area, a place labeled not just as a "hotspot" that was named the worst parish in Jamaica, I strive to heal and make a difference.

We seek to be prepared for opportunities to educate our children. Van went on to the University of Technology. She was assisted by family members. She also travels overseas for the student work-study programme. This was useful in providing much-needed funds for her school fees. Ron, our second daughter, went to the Caribbean Maritime Institute. She was also assisted by family members as well as the student work-travel programme overseas.

Rom accepted the invitation to attend Northern Caribbean University (NCU) on their work-study programme. This became a reality because someone was at the right place at the right time. Opportunity favors the prepared. At one of the community interventions in York Town, an initiative of the collaboration between the Jamaica Constabulary Force (JCF) Chaplaincy Unit and the NCU Department of Behavioural and Social Sciences, Dr. Grace Kelly shared the range of programmes available at the NCU. She further extended an appeal that there is an opportunity to help a needy student who has left high school, with subjects and can be a role model for his or her community. The community members shouted in a chorus, "Romario Pusey." A volunteer rode a cycle to the construction site where he was working and brought him to the function. The following Monday, Romario was on the NCU campus. Many persons mentored and supported him, including Dr. Pauline Gayle-Bettne and Dr. Grace. He was also a recipient of the NCU RESCUE 2020 programme (Restoring Every Student's Confidence Using Education), an initiative of President Lincoln Edwards. After four years, he graduated with his Bachelor's degree.

It was a joy to have more social and emotional support once my wife, Kathleeen, returned home. This was a real joy for me just to have her home. Normally, I had to prepare the meals and do the laundry but now that she is back, I was relieved of these chores. I was more able to talk and share intimate conversations, which gave me good feelings and boosted my self-esteem.

I accepted my situation by putting my mind to my condition, and kept reminding myself that one day, I will walk again. It took eight years for this to be a reality. The year 2019 brought much joy. I put away my stick on the doctor's order. That week I was lucky; all the clinics I attended gave me a clean walking discharge.

In this situation, I am grateful that God has prepared me to go through my trials. It was heart-rending but I stood the test of time. I am a conqueror and I don't have to ask Why me Lord. It was just a test and I know I am victorious. Living in a volatile community would have shaped my emotional experience and dictated the order of the day. I live each day by consciously determining that I will bloom where I have been planted like a beautiful lily in a muddy pond. Personally, life has new meaning each day and I seek to share them along the way. I reflect on the days, weeks, months, and years when I was unable to walk and my mind would get into a negative gear, but those moments would be short lived because I clinged to the belief that I would walk again. I was injured physically and this strengthened me mentally. Just as I have learned to walk a second time, I have learned to nurture positive thoughts and feelings. Forgiveness has helped me to appreciate the smaller things of life. I am able to enjoy life regardless of my challenges.

When I consider my journey to walking again and how far I have traveled, the mingling thoughts did not bother me much since I was moving.

Sometimes I would be tired of staying inside the house, so I would go on the outside stand by the gate and look around. Being in the fresh air provides better concentration and makes me feel happy within myself. This has enabled me to demonstrate a better appreciation for nature and the smaller blessings of life.

To every reader who has experienced scars like mine, do not stop there and do not allow those scars to limit what you can achieve. You are a star and you must continue to shine brilliantly; you can be a star from your scar! Having used my experience with my scars, praying has helped me tremendously. It has aided my mental healing, and comfort, and I am able to fulfill my purpose. I have done it and so can you. Push ahead, never stop, and you will be victorious.

I want to share the message of restoration and forgiveness. This story is just a starting point in sharing my journey of trials to triumph and as the story gets into the library of your hearts; it will emancipate fear, stimulate forgiveness, and brighten the path for emotional healing. My will is to preach the message of forgiveness to the members of my community; by doing this, I hope to contribute to a more caring and responsible community. I will continue to use my story to help others who have been impacted by violence to move on from trials to triumphs.

If you have been scarred because of situations in life and didn't have an opportunity to tell your story to others, a knockdown is real; you can overcome by praying, pushing, and talking to trustworthy persons who understand or may also have been through scars of their own. God knows your pain and He knows your scars. You just have to put your trust in Him to make it better. Every setback in life is a setup to a comeback.

STEPS TOWARDS INTENTIONAL HEALING

These action steps are designed to help you intentionally navigate your scars. I hope you will find them useful.

Prepare for Opportunities: Whatever you are going through, look out for opportunities as well. Although you are going through your difficulties, grasp opportunities as they knock and make good use of them. You don't have to wait until the bad times pass before you start to live… live through the bad times while you prepare for the good.

Increase Social Support: Your social network is of vital importance; no man is an island and no man stands alone. Family and friends are good sources of support, as they can provide the medicine that will help you heal socially and emotionally. When you are feeling down, you will need someone with whom you can share, and laugh. You should never run out of social support, so keep family members and friends close to your heart; they can even surprise you with quality support.

Self Will: Accept your situation by putting your mind to the condition. This is a powerful step that can work for the good of everyone who is willing to do it. Don't be angry, but rather channel your energy into developing the self-will to push forward while accepting your situation. Tell yourself that you can do it and make it happen. Never give up.

In my situation, I was blessed to have a mediator, Dr. Grace Kelly, who taught me the way forward, that life can be what you want, and that praying and asking God for intervention can transform your life. She taught me to believe in myself and focus on my purpose on earth. I invite you to do the same and when you are absent from this life, your legacy will still motivate others and your children. Have faith, persevere, have goodwill, and receive the blessings of God. Amen.

CHAPTER 28

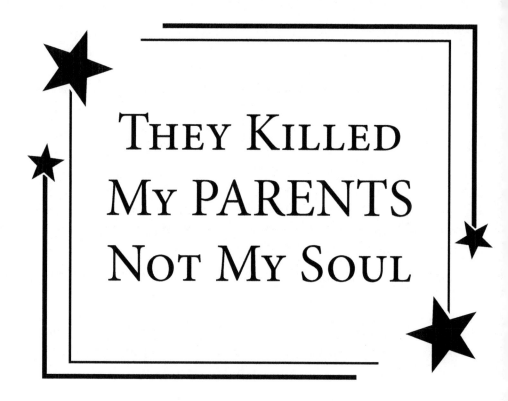

THEY KILLED MY PARENTS NOT MY SOUL

BY: **DR. MARIE CLAUDINE MUKAMABANO**

Dr. Marie Claudine Mukamabano

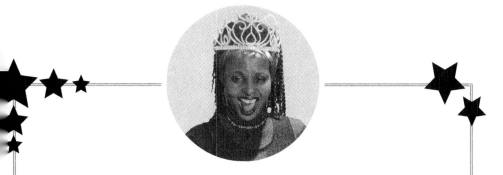

"They killed my parents, but they couldn't KILL my Soul. Only God, who created my soul, has the power to KILL it. I became a teenage orphan, but I continued to LIVE." - MUKAMABANO (2022)

An International Awards Winning Author who won the 2019 Global Humanitarian Award in Geneva, Europe for using ICT Information Communication Technology to Change Lives, Dr. Claudine MUKAMABANOis Founder of WHY DO I EXIST? KUKI NDIHO? With Mission to Heal and Empower Orphans after becoming a Rwandan orphaned teenage survivor herself, she refused to be just a victim, but became victorious and forgave the killers of her parents. Dr. Claudine is the author of The Power of Social Media: Be Yourself & Change Somebody's Life Today! and an upcoming book she named Bank for Orphans, which narrates how she gives the opportunity to people of good will to financially contribute to help Rwandan Young Adults Orphans and most Vulnerable Single Mothers in spirit of leave no one behind to create income generating activities by becoming entrepreneurs. She is founder and CEO of Why Do I Exist? and Kuki Ndiho Rwanda Orphans Support Project. Dr. Claudine works every day to honor her promise to God of helping Rwandan orphans which she vowed during the genocide against Tutsi in Rwanda when she was running for her life jumping over the bodies of people, thinking that she was the next to be killed. She said, "Lord if you save my life and I survive, I will help orphans." Then my voice inside of her head asked, "How are you going to help orphans when your childhood dream is to study Math and get a Ph.D. in Mathematics and Science?"She quickly replied to that voice, "I will study Business and make money and help orphans instead of getting Ph.D. in Mathematics."

INTENTION

You have the power inside of you and the ability to heal your wounded heart. Do not wait for those who wounded your heart to pity you and come to rescue and save you. Take responsibility for your own healing and take refuge in God, your Creator, and ask His Majesty to help you heal. Remember healing takes time, courage, dedication and commitment, so listen to your heart, take action, and implement your ideas of healing yourself. Focus on mainly doing things you love. Avoid those who hurt you or remind you of the pain, especially in your fragile moments, as in those moments your healing journey can be easily sabotaged.

THEY KILLED MY PARENTS NOT MY SOUL

As a child, I was full of joy with my lovely mother who often encouraged me to dance at all times because she knew that I loved to dance. I was a happy little girl. Mom would call me each time she heard a beautiful song on the radio and every time she called me, I would dance for her. Sometimes, I would dance for her in front of her guests; I didn't mind who was in the house. My mom told me to dance and immediately I would create a stage and start dancing like nobody's business. I would dance with such precision, energy, and excitement like I was entering a world famous dance competition with millions of people from around the world watching. After dancing, my mother used to give me sweet treats to eat or Fanta to drink as an incentive. Then she would instruct me to go back where I was.

I even remember, like it was yesterday, one of the good memories from my childhood. I was under five years old. I was jolly, jumping around making noise while my mother was sitting with some of the women from the community having their conversation. I overheard one of them saying to my mother, "You should beat your child and make her sit down and be quiet." My mother replied, "Leave my daughter alone. I know my daughter and she is very smart. Even if I should die today, of all my children, I know she will survive and make a living." I said, "Mom, tell them, tell them."

I grew up believing that I could do anything because I had a supportive mother who had my back. I had my Creator who wanted everything beautiful and good for me. I was very happy, joyful, full of life and peace of mind, and focused on my dream projects from an early age.

Life never really knocked me down because I believe that life does not exist without me. Horrible life circumstances destroyed my family when I was but a little girl. I was exposed to the stench and gruesome realities of dying, death, and decay the day my parents were killed. When my family was killed, I recognised quickly that my life was in my hands now. In one sudden moment, I had become my own father and my own mother with no auntie, no uncle, and no grandparents. I was suddenly ALONE! I became the one who had to figure out what to do with my life, bad, ugly or good. I became a teenage orphan, but I continued to live.

My mother had introduced me to the Creator of the Universe when she was alive. So, in the delicate crevices of my childhood mind, I knew that even though they killed my parents, they couldn't KILL my Soul. Only God, who created my soul and spirit, has the power to KILL it. So, I have lived with the knowledge that only God has that power to destroy the soul and because He is, I can live.

So, even though horrible, very sad, and hurtful things have happened in my life, I tell myself, "That is the reality of the life I am living in and everything will be up to me."

I navigated from scars to be a star by having faith in God and in myself, forcing myself to learn more about God's promises, and making them personal. I pray to God from that space with a full understanding. I have immersed myself into trusting God and He has kept His promises because He is not a man that He should lie (Numbers 33:19, KJV). By His hands only, in 2005, chosen among 600 applicants from around the world, I won a scholarship to come to New York City. By His grace, I also kept my promise to my people.

INTENTIONAL HEALING: FROM SCARS TO STARS

In December 2013, I organized and hosted Trauma Healing Training in Kigali, Rwanda to benefit genocide survivors. One of the experts I invited to help and teach my orphans came to Rwanda from New Jersey. She is a Jewish American who I met on Facebook in October of the same year, 2013. In November, she came to my office on Madison Avenue in Manhattan, New York City. Then in December, she flew to Rwanda for the training titled How to Overcome Trauma. I used Facebook to promote and invite genocide survivors to attend the Trauma Healing Training program. I was amazed to see many people who wanted to join the training in Kigali. In promoting the training, I shared how they will benefit from the training and what survivors of genocide need to know about trauma. I also learned about the importance of storytelling, music, and dance at New York University, where I graduated from International Trauma Studies with professors at Columbia and NYU Universities. The successful outcome and mindset shifts from genocide orphan survivors who attended the Trauma Healing in Kigali inspired me to write The Power Of Social Media. I believe social media is a gift God gave humankind; it's up to me and you to take advantage of it.

So, instead of complaining or being revengeful, I am using the power of social media to position myself and change somebody's life by lighting the path for other Orphan survivors to see more clearly how to navigate their scars. Today! I got an epiphany from God to write a book to share my experience and how other changemakers can benefit and leverage the power of social media to achieve their dream goals in a short period of time. Being a part of this anthology Intentional Healing: From Scars to Stars is the beginning of another journey more healing to my people.

I help people create good, positive memories by creating more joyful memories to remember all the time instead of only remembering bad memories. I did not focus on my pain. If you focus on the pain, you create more pain. I wish I could tell you differently, but I am sharing with you my own life experiences. That is how I managed to navigate my painful life experiences. I always give thanks to my Creator, who protected me during the genocide in Rwanda. His Majesty helped me to fulfill my promise of helping Rwandan orphans.

Today, I confess to tell you that my Creator protected me and He also helped me fulfill my heart's desire of helping Rwandan orphans through my charitable Organization Kuki Ndiho? which means, "Why do I exist?" During a Mother's Day celebration in New Jersey in May

2019, God also took it to the next level when He reminded me to create and establish a Bank For Orphans which was my original dream project idea. This reminder fuelled the establishment of the bank which is fully functional today. At the Bank For Orphans, we teach orphans to develop their dreams into big ideas, set goals, and work towards achieving them through employment or entrepreneurship. The bank also lends adult orphans capital to start and sustain their businesses as they change their lives and the lives of their next generation. At the Bank For Orphans, we also teach adult orphans how to dream big and take action toward achieving their big dream! We teach them that success leaves clues as such it is very important that they leave footprints in the sand of time that other orphans can learn from as they build a legacy for themselves, their families, and by extension, the world at large.

My pain has fuelled my passion and my purpose. I salute all the amazing people who care for orphans around the world and those who support my charity to be where I am today. I dedicate this story to the orphans I have helped as well as those who will benefit from my work in the future, as well as my siblings. The fact that I am alive is very important. I give thanks to my Creator every day because only people who are alive can give thanks with our physical lives. Integrity and loving life help more people who need my support, especially Rwandan orphans working every day to promote peace. I share my story to inspire others.

There is a saying that "hurt people, hurt people." From my theistic worldview, this statement is not really 100% true because not all hurt people hurt others; in fact, from my experience, most hurt people love to help others, promoting peace and creating opportunities to help others overcome what we have already overcome. As someone who has experienced hurt, I have focused on helping others to live a joyful lifestyle. I spend time teaching them how to forgive and the value of forgiveness. For those of us who are Christians, we see forgiveness not as an option, but as an obligation because Jesus came to show us God's mercy and unconditional forgiveness.

The commitment I made the day I was skipping over dead bodies to a place of safety lives on through my charity and my online campaigns which are powered through social media. This will continue to be at the forefront of my mind and my business ventures as this Rwandan orphan continues to live on.

STEPS TOWARDS INTENTIONAL HEALING

Have Faith in God and in Yourself. Force yourself to learn more about God's promises, make them personal, and pray to God from a space of full understanding. Trust that God keeps His promises because He is not a human being.

Do Movements. Engage in activities you love. Dance! I love to dance! Do more of what you love to do and create high level vibration and frequency because more joy helps to overpower pain. When you embrace this approach, you will create joyful memories to remember instead of mostly remembering bad memories. If you only focus on your pain, you create more pain.

Listen to and Obey Your Heart. Your heart knows what's best for you and your heart loves you so much! Be reminded that the God who created you loves you beyond measure no matter what. you are loved and protected, so act like it.

Forgive Quickly! Forgiveness helps us to speed up our healing process. Forgiveness is an expression of God's beauty. When you forgive, you automatically access the wisdom, healing, and creativities, gifts, talents, and powers of God. All you want from God is all hiding in forgiveness.

Focus On Being Grateful. Focus on being grateful, give thanks, and don't complain because it brings you more things to complain about, causing you to feel down without any reason. When you focus on being grateful, giving thanks to God for life, it opens many doors and you start to see how you can use your pain to empower yourself and tell your story to help others who may be going through something similar or exactly what you experienced.

RESOURCES

Instagram: doctorclaudinevictorious

Facebook: marieclaudine.mukamabano

Clubhouse: drClaudineM

CHAPTER 29

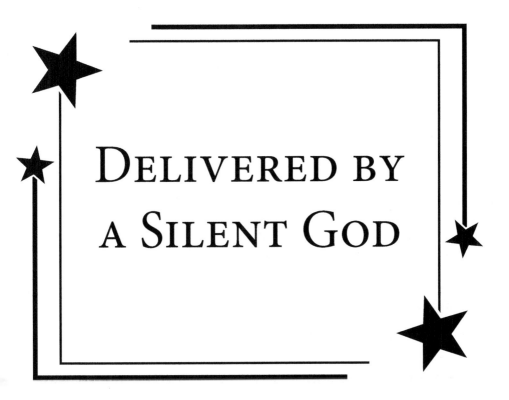

DELIVERED BY
A SILENT GOD

BY: SASHOI GRANT

INTENTIONAL HEALING: FROM SCARS TO STARS

SASHOI GRANT

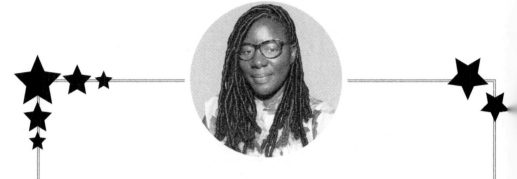

"If God's not with it, I don't want it." - Sashoi Grant
"Be anxious for nothing, but in everything by prayer and
supplication, with thanksgiving, let your requests be made known
to God; and the peace of God, which surpasses all understanding,
will guard your hearts and minds through Christ Jesus." -
Philippians 4:6,7 (NIV)

Sashoi M. Grant was born and raised on the beautiful island of Jamaica. She has over 20 years of experience serving individuals with disabilities. Sashoi began her career as a Direct Support Professional at New York Foundling (NYF). While at NYF she obtained her degree in nursing and became a licensed registered nurse and started her career in nursing. She was later promoted to Assistant Nursing Supervisor and subsequently Vice President of Nursing. Within her current role, Sashoi is responsible to create quality nursing indicators that ensure person-centered and highest quality of care. She is a Seventh Day Adventist Christian who is actively involved in her church and heads the Health and Temperance and Community Service departments. Her deep passion for youth ministries led her to serve as a Bronx Area Coordinator for the Greater New York Conference of Seventh Day Adventist. Sashoi loves to paint, cook vegan dishes, and enjoys nature. Her mission is to bring joy to anyone that she comes in contact with while being Jesus' hands and feet.

INTENTION

I want others to know that God is real. He is sometimes quiet during some dark areas of our lives, and it causes us to question if He really exists. Be encouraged, for He is right there with you. Our challenges promote growth and it's in those moments when we are feeling alone that we learn to put our trust in God. God is the source of wisdom and knowledge. He has equipped doctors to assist us with our physical and mental health. When you encounter mental health challenges, never be afraid to enlist the aid of a psychologist or counselor.

DELIVERED BY A SILENT GOD

I can remember the laughter and fun I had from being around my family. It was summer time and my nieces and nephews were visiting. My family is comedic in nature and so there was never a dull moment when they were around. Laughter mixed with the smell of my mother's cooking provided all the love and comfort I needed. The love we shared was palpable and soothing to the soul.

The restrictions of the pandemic were being lifted, and I was able to socialize more with my family and friends. The isolation was becoming a thing of the past and it was time to reconnect in person. Brunch in the city with my friends was my favorite thing to do. Nothing beats good company, good food, and good vibes. Whenever I wanted to relax, I would paint or just go to one of my happy places. My happy place is anywhere in nature preferably by a body of water. The ripple of the water and the gentle swaying of the trees often ushered me into a quiet rest. Nature has a way of calming me and allowing me to slow down from the hustle and bustle of life.

I had my circle of sisters who were always supportive and they were always available whenever I needed a prayer and words of encouragement. In-person church was back in progress and it was so refreshing to actually go back to church and enjoy true fellowship with my church family. I was in a job that I loved, even with its many stressors. There was so much to give God thanks for. I had worked on myself through therapy and was more comfortable in my own skin. I had learned to set healthy boundaries and started seeing myself the way God saw me. I was enjoying life, feeling free, and self-sufficient. I was really feeling good knowing that I was loved and meant so much to others. Life was good and every day I woke up thankful to God for all His provisions and for waking me up in my right mind.

One night, I stayed up late listening to an influencer. The content was nothing that would enhance personal or spiritual growth, but it was sensational. I fell asleep to the voice of the influencer just going on and on. At approximately 2:00 A.M., I jumped out of my sleep and I was in a state of panic. I did not have a bad dream, so I was puzzled by the state of panic I was in. I jumped out of bed and I felt like the darkness of the night was closing in on me. I ran to the front door to escape what I was experiencing and realized that it was the dead at night. I was shaking, my heart was pounding, and I felt like there was impending doom. I have Sickle Cell disease, and I am prescribed Percocet to address painful crises. I had a bottle on my desk; I looked at it and surprisingly thought of taking the entire bottle just to get some relief. My senses kicked in, and I thought to myself that I would have killed myself if I took that route. I quickly took a Benadryl tablet. I ran to my room and shut the influencer off and went to YouTube to find videos with Bible verses to calm me down. I got back in bed and fell asleep to Bible verses being played. At that point I realized that by spending so much time on social media, and listening to different personalities, I have given so many random people access to my mind. The next morning when I woke up, I started to think about the events that occurred hours before. I realized that I almost committed suicide without even thinking about it. I have always been claustrophobic and did not like enclosed areas such as elevators, airplanes, or trains. Whenever I experienced any of those situations, my escape would be to go out in an open area. However, this time I felt trapped in the world and the sky was enclosing me. I thought to myself,

INTENTIONAL HEALING: FROM SCARS TO STARS

"Sashoi this cannot become a thing; if you feel stuck in the world, where is your escape?" At this moment, an open space was as claustrophobic as an elevator.

The darkness of the night seemed to envelop me and I felt like I was going to die. My heart pounded and my head felt as if it was going to burst open. I was paralyzed by fear and I could not stop the thoughts in my mind. I did what I always did when I had trouble in my life: I went to God. I knew he would be able to help me. I prayed and asked God to help me, but my prayers seemed to be strangled by the darkness of which I became afraid. I didn't feel safe anymore at night. I felt like the house was going to cave in on me and I would die under the rubble. After a night of battling with fear and anxiety, I would fall asleep at daybreak and I would wake up feeling like I was battered and beaten. I suffered alone; I did not want to disclose what I was experiencing to anyone because I did not want to end up in a psychiatric hospital. One thing for sure was that I did not want to depend on medications for my mental well-being. I had become a walking panic attack. I showed up at work and I performed my duties while experiencing internal turmoil. One day, I jokingly asked the psychologist at work if I could use her couch. She smiled and said, "You are welcome anytime." I wrestled with telling her, but I was too afraid of being seen as unable to carry out my job responsibilities. My circle of sisters and mother did not know. They prayed, but their prayers were not specific because they did not know the details.

Gripped by the hands of anxiety, I longed for emancipation day. I prostrated before God in my bedroom and pleaded with Him to deliver me, but was met by silence. I was distressed; however I still prayed as in my own warped way I believed. I knew the power of my God and that He was able to deliver me from anxiety. A friend connected me with a Christian therapist who helped me to process my thoughts and navigate my way through the darkest hour of my life. My therapy sessions also provided me with tools to redirect my thoughts and pointed me to the one who was able to help me. I found Bible promises that I could claim, such as, Isaiah 43:2 (KJV), "When thou passest through the waters, I will be with thee; and through the rivers, they shall not overflow thee: when thou walkest through the fire, thou shalt not be burned; neither shall the flame kindle upon thee." These promises reassured me that I could depend on God and that I was not alone. I learned to rely on God more fully to guide and protect me. Being vulnerable with people in my inner circle was a means of comfort and support. I no longer hid my thoughts and fears, so they were able to encourage me and help me have a more positive outlook. I felt God's presence; even in His silence, and knew I was loved.

I continued to integrate my prayer, therapy sessions, and the support of my inner circle, and I was slowly able to make progress by replacing fear with faith. Timidity gave way to boldness and confidence in God as the murky waters of anxiety gave rise to flowers of hope, peace, and joy.

Doubts, fear, and some amount of concern clogged my mind. Why wasn't I trusting God? For every question of this kind, I was reminded through a personal life experience to trust God more. In my first session with my new therapist, she prayed and then I proceeded to tell her my issues. Her prayer made a difference, and it calmed my fears. Every activity she gave reinforced my need to trust God. Why talk to her? Why complete the activities? These were all answered through the realization that they each helped me. Journaling helped me with anxiety and made me appreciate the power of prayer. Why pray? This was answered through my new lens, and it was a source of strength that quelled my fears. During this time, what seemed to be the worst season of my life was actually my darkest hour before my new day. I often asked myself where was God in my darkest hour. This question was answered when I was reminded that He kept me alive and provided for me. My thoughts were telling me that I was unsafe and that death was near, but my reality was that the Sovereign God was with me and I was safe.

I was literally fighting for my life. It was a life or death situation, and I was determined to choose life. Choosing life forced me to depend on the only one who was able to deliver me. This experience has deepened my relationship with God and has taught me how to truly trust Him.

You never appreciate a good night's sleep until you've experienced insomnia. Night after night I went to bed and God gave me sweet sleep. Day by day, God was working on me; slowly, anxiety and panic attacks were of the past. Though God was silent in my situation, I now see how He was orchestrating my deliverance. First with the change in my insurance, which allowed me to connect with a Christian therapist. The therapist He used pointed me back to Him. She challenged me to put my trust in God. She showed me how I was taking on God's role in trying to be in control. She reminded me that God could rescue me from any situation in which I may feel trapped. I started to slowly let go and left the future in the hands of a Sovereign God.

God is not done writing my story, and He is still molding and fashioning me for His glory. I am now intentional about guarding my mental health and making self-care a priority. I have decided that I will not worry over the things I cannot control, but I will show up every day and put my best foot forward. I am reassured that even in His silence, His deliverance is deafening. Telling my story has been instrumental in my healing process, and I will continue to echo His goodness to any and everyone who is willing to listen. I am living my best life in Christ by the daily baptism of the Holy Spirit. This comes with a peace that is beyond my imagination, a more intimate relationship with God, and faith that is anchored in Him. My Abba is taking me on a journey from fear to faith and I am enjoying the ride. The ride will not be without bumps and obstacles, but with Him I need not be afraid. With God and my therapist, I can smile at the storm.

Philippians 4:6-7 (KJV) says, "Be careful for nothing; but in everything by prayer and supplication with thanksgiving let your requests be made known unto God. And the peace of God, which passeth all understanding, shall keep your hearts and minds through Christ Jesus." 1 Peter 5:6-7 (KJV) says, "Humble yourselves therefore under the mighty hand of God, that he may exalt you in due time: Casting all your care upon him; for he careth for you." These texts have been helpful in my healing process. I taped them to my laptop, so I am constantly reminded of God's promises. God is telling us not to worry about anything. He wants us to take all our problems to Him so that he can give us peace. Peace that allows you to live in a world of chaos, without being bothered because you know who is in control. Stand on God's promises, for they are sure.

STEPS TOWARDS INTENTIONAL HEALING

Your deliverance from your circumstance is nearer than you think. You just need to be intentional and drink from your CUP.

Create a community. Human beings are social creatures, so we function best as a part of a community. A problem shared is a problem halved. When you engage your community, you will have a support system to encourage you. They will become your personal cheerleaders who will help you believe that you can make it. Their support will be a source of strength. As you tap into your support system, you will find that your feelings of anxiety will lose the stronghold that they once had in your life. They will fade as your strengthened character shines through.

Utilize a therapist. A good therapist helps you to verbalize your thoughts so that you can analyze them and become more empowered. The liberation that you feel as you are freed from shame enables you to use the resources that are available to you. This also creates a safe space where you can be vulnerable in a nonjudgmental place that facilitates emotional wellness and healing.

Pray about your situation. Have a heart-to-heart conversation with God. Tears are a language that God interprets. Your emotional nakedness with God will open the door for Him to act on your behalf. I am living testimony that God moves in silence. Prayer puts you in direct connection with a Sovereign God who is in control. He has all the solutions to your problems even before you become aware of them. When in connection with Him, you will be connected with a Source of strength and power that is stronger than anything you will ever have to face.

RESOURCES

Linktree: https://linktr.ee/sassyshoi

Instagram: Sassyshoi

Facebook: Sashoi Grantl

CHAPTER 30

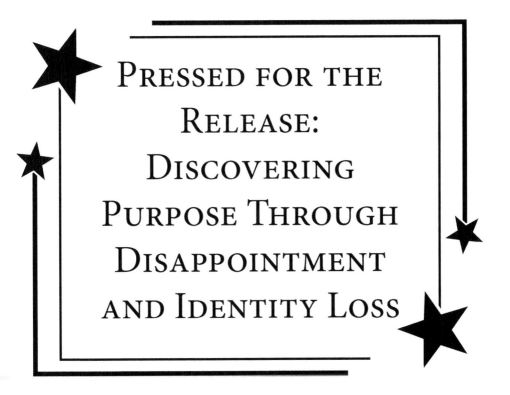

PRESSED FOR THE RELEASE: DISCOVERING PURPOSE THROUGH DISAPPOINTMENT AND IDENTITY LOSS

BY: **DR. KEISHA ANN THOMAS**

Dr. Keisha Ann Thomas

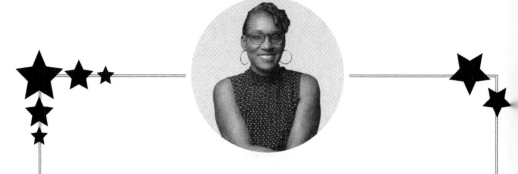

"No pain should be wasted."
- Keisha Thomas (2022)

Keisha Ann Thomas, D.Sc., MBA., B.Sc, MO., is a woman predestined for the empowerment and wellness of other women, on a life journey that was designed to equip her with the wisdom and the experience she will need to effectively answer that call.

A mother to three beautiful girls, Dr. Keisha Thomas lives each day intentionally, in hope that ultimately, she will have laid the right foundation to raise empowered women. She is a self-employed Marketing Consultant at F.E.M. Events and Marketing Consultancy, with more than twenty years' experience in media sales and marketing; a strategist and repositioning expert with a strong track record spanning both the private and the public sector.

Dr. Thomas has a first degree in Business Administration (Marketing Major) from the University of the Caribbean (UCC, now the University of the Commonwealth Caribbean); A Master of Business Administration (Marketing Major) from the University of Technology (Utech) and has recently completed her Doctor of Communication Degree with the Atlantic International University (AIU) in the USA. She is the Founder and Executive Director of Predestined, a registered charity for the empowerment and wellness of women. She is an Associate Pastor and a licensed Marriage Officer of the Island of Jamaica.

Intention

It is my prayer that anyone who reads my story will walk away with the understanding that there is no place that life can take you where you cannot find your way back. Life is a journey full of uncertainties, with hills and valleys called victories and disappointments, but though the journey may take us on unanticipated paths, with a sense of self-awareness and God's divine guidance, we will always find purpose. Know who you are, and you will eventually find your way home.

Pressed for the Release: Discovering Purpose Through Disappointment and Identity Loss

As soon as we are old enough to dream, we begin to form concepts of who we believe we are destined to become and how great our lives should be. We never learn early enough that God really has the final say. I grew up in a very poor family. We were never able to afford most things, but the one thing we had in abundance was love. We were amazingly close. Our parents got married as teenage sweethearts. We knew they loved each other, and they loved us; although we were poor, we believed that with the help of God and the love and support of each other, we had enough to make it. We were the Bailey family, resilient and strong.

Mommy accepted the Lord at age twenty-one and with many episodes of rebellion and mischief in between, Daddy met the Lord six years later. We had a strong Christian foundation as eventually, they would pastor a ministry together. They were inseparable. You never saw one without the other. As children, we admired their marriage so much; it was a common aspiration among the five of us. When we weren't dreaming of elaborate professions to lift us out of poverty, we were fantasizing about marrying the person of our dreams so we could experience the joys of romance and beautiful families such as the one we grew up in. At age twenty-two, I was walking down the aisle in a beautiful Saturday morning wedding ceremony, and I was a beautiful June bride. The wedding happened only two days after my final college exams. We were so in love.

By the time my husband and I got married, my parents were establishing a marriage ministry in our local church, and I knew that was the place for me to serve. We became the resident planners and organizers of the Annual Marriage Retreats. We organized every marriage event, and we were great at finding resource persons: psychologists, psychotherapists, sex therapists, marriage counsellors and entertainment. Whatever we thought the couples needed to keep the fire of love burning, we sourced it. I was a creative event planner who came alive for these marriage and family enrichment events. For me, it was ministry, and so for more than seventeen years, we served our church organization in this capacity. I was soon ready to pursue my Doctoral Degree in Marriage and Family Therapy, willing to spend the rest of my life giving back and pouring into others. What we had was real and my passion was real. Those who knew us admired us until one day we weren't that couple anymore and a new chapter of life began.

My husband and I found ourselves challenged in our own marriage. We were headed for a divorce after twenty-two years of marriage with three beautiful daughters. We were losing the battle to our own marital conflicts and with that, we lost the respect and admiration from others. As soon as our challenges became somewhat obvious to those around us, we began to be marginalized, distanced from those we once served and ministered to in so many ways. It was as though a struggling marriage was now spiritually contagious. We spent years serving others, but now the doctor had become the patient. Other than our family members, and the very, very few close friends we had, those who supported us did so from a distance with prayer. We certainly appreciated the prayers, but I couldn't help but notice the absence of fellowship, the lifeline that we had offered so many other struggling marriages for so many years. It was as though we wore the proverbial bell, while shouting "unclean." The whispers were loud and always somehow found their way into my spirit.

Once our struggle became evident, we lost our authenticity, irrelevant to those who once listened to us. For as long as we were navigating our own challenges, persons distanced themselves from us, seemingly in an effort to protect their own marriages. The message was clear. We had lost the respect of the other couples, and with that, their fellowship and support.

While going through my own storms trying desperately to keep my head above water, I felt God leading me to stand in the gap for other women who were hurting from similar challenges. I was being pressed and being cured like an olive freshly picked and ready to be preserved. I was being squeezed to dispel the bitterness that would not linger at the expense of the olive's exotic taste. I resigned my media job and started hosting empowerment conferences and transformational retreats for distressed, discontented women or those simply in need of a support network to help them pull through life's difficult moments. We were still fighting to save our marriage and family. There was brokenness all around: a broken marriage, a broken family, broken home and broken hearts, yet in 2018, I officially launched, Predestined, for the Empowerment and Wellness of Women. Participants at our functions reported that they got a fresh start, a new beginning. I pulled strength from every event, but the miracle I longed for was never to be received.

When the divorce began, I found myself in a predicament. I was experiencing loss such as I never imagined. We had lost the fight that many others had won with our help. I felt like a failure. I could not save our own family, not even for our daughters' sake and I had to accept this defeat and gracefully bow out. The happy nuclear family was no more. I was now a single mother of three. I had literally been married for exactly half of my life when the divorce started, and I built my world around being a wife and a mother. I prided myself on who I was in my marriage, my family, and my church, more than anything else. I could no longer appreciate the person in the mirror. My childhood never prepared me for this, coming from a rich history of strong marriages. My great grandparents were married for sixty-five years, and this legacy continued through the generations in my aunts and uncles and my dear parents. I had spent the last twenty-two years building on this legacy, but I was now helplessly watching it all crumble and my sense of purpose was crumbling with it. I had lost my identity to a broken marriage and family.

Life became complicated. I was no longer doing the thing that brought me the greatest gratification. And where was I to go now and what was I to do with the rest of my life? I no longer felt accepted where I once dominated. I was experiencing rejection where I once served. Confused and bewildered, I had no idea who I had become. I was trying to be strong for my girls but the little girl inside me had gone back to sucking her thumb. My insecurities were heightened. I felt lost and scared. I was grieving.

Moving through the stages of grief, there were days when I was in denial, wondering if I was dreaming. This could not be happening. I was hurting for so long that now I was simply numb. When I had the capacity to feel anything at all, it was anger. I was angry at my circumstances and I was sometimes angry at God. I had lost control and that was something to which I was unaccustomed. I was a planner, organizer, administrator, and manager. Losing control was not a thing. I was facing shame, overthinking everything, and of course wondering if there was anything else I could have done that would have changed the outcome. I wanted to believe I didn't just fail. I was fighting depression so I kept my hands busy with not a moment to spare. I was serving in the pastoral capacity while holding a full-time job and mothering my girls through the crisis. I was forced to accept the truth that it was out of my hands. There was nothing I could have done to change my circumstances and I had to own my new life.

In search of fresh validation, I got certified as a Transformational Life Coach. I was now ready to finally pursue my Doctoral degree, but I had no idea what area to study as my dream of studying Psychology and becoming a Licensed Marriage and Family Therapist seemed irrelevant having lost the marriage that validated me. I had forgotten the love I had for marketing and communication and how naturally gifted I was in this field. I sat in the parking lot in my vehicle one day and the tears flooded my face like a river which had broken its banks. Distressed and bewildered, I remember praying to God for direction. I was scared for my relevance. I asked the Lord for direction. I could not emotionally handle studies in family therapy at that juncture, but I was also scared of walking in another direction. I asked God to speak to me with undeniable clarity on what my Doctoral studies should be in. After returning from my lunch break, about fifteen minutes after settling in at my desk, I received a call from my CEO. As I closed the door of her office behind me, she proceeded to speak into my destiny.

INTENTIONAL HEALING: FROM SCARS TO STARS

I had been struggling with unanswered questions. What was the purpose of my experience in planning, organizing, and interacting with the couples if I was unable to serve in that area anymore? I was an influencer but for what purpose? And how would I use this experience and my competencies now? Without her knowing it, the words my CEO spoke resuscitated my spirit and gave me direction. She said, "Know who you are and who you are supposed to be." She further said, "I don't think you know how brilliant and naturally talented you are." She proceeded to share with me that based on my natural talent and personality, I should be groomed to become a senior communication personnel for the Agency and commissioned me to research the possibilities. Upon leaving her office that day, I knew God had instantly answered my prayer. I went home that evening and immediately submitted my application for a Doctoral Degree in Communication. In that moment I realized nothing I had been through would ever be wasted. There was purpose in every experience. I was grateful that my life had prepared me for a place I had never been. Two years later in 2022, I completed that degree and realized that Keisha Ann Thomas is a woman Predestined for Women's Empowerment and Wellness. My experiences were equipping me to speak life into their troubled circumstances.

My charity is now officially registered in a second country as I seek opportunities to communicate hope to women as they navigate hardships. I am thankful that I am able to see the power behind my pain and I am grateful for those who continue to help me navigate my difficult experiences without losing my identity.

It was so much easier for me to become bitter rather than better when traversing the streets of life's pains, but I could not effectively and sincerely serve others if bitterness prevailed. I continue to undergo processing of the harshest form, as olives cured with lye or caustic soda components are typically one of the more delectable kinds. I thought that in pouring into other marriages I was also ensuring mine was anchored securing a kind of Godly reward for the good deeds done; but life is not necessarily fair, and I learnt to still celebrate the victories of others even in the face of personal loss. It is the reason service to others still positively influences my own healing process. Bake me first a cake, said the prophet to the widow. My own healing is buried in the healing of others, a purpose bigger than the pain I've carried.

I have become deliberate about guarding my values in defense of who I am, knowing that hurt unattended has the ability to steal my identity. I have also sought professional guidance on my journey to intentional healing. Despite my loss, my conviction remains the same: Marriage is honourable in all things, and the bed is undefiled.

There are two types of hurting people in this world; the first type spends their lives avenging themselves, ensuring everyone else suffers as much as they did. The second type spends their lives trying to prevent others from having to ever experience their pain. I am the second type. I understand now that my knowledge and experience are valuable, and my pain could bring healing to someone else. I may one day in the distant future, return to the pursuit of a marriage and family therapy career, but for now, as I pursue my own healing, I find life in helping other women find their way through the very things that challenged me. After all, what good is pain if we never discover its true purpose?

Today, my women's empowerment organization is anchored in the principle of women who have been through stuff, reaching back to pull another woman through. The reality is that without the right kind of support, someone else could fall under the burdens we overcome. I am determined to continue healing my scars and shine as the star I am destined to be and light the path for others behind.

The truth is that we often make the mistake of defining ourselves by the challenges we face or the things we acquire when in fact, we are none of those things. Neither are we what we have been through. Our experiences are meant to prepare us for service in one way or another. I am not my training, though it has enhanced my life. Neither are we what we own because assets, possessions, positions, and careers may all be lost, and our status in life can change in a moment, but if we know who we were before those things, we may somehow find the motivation to rebuild. A person who knows his or her identity, will always find the way back to hope. Do you know who you are? Do you know and claim your purpose and destiny? Will you take the time to preserve that legacy and be the best version of yourself?

Steps Towards Intentional Healing

Here are three things in which strength can be found as intentionally transitioned from 'scars to stars,' and trust that you may find hope through these practical tips:

Firstly, accept failure as a time-bound experience and not a permanent state. Failure is a necessary part of any training, as it challenges us to improve on who we are and what we have in order to conquer the same test tomorrow. It highlights the opportunity for growth and development in a particular area of interest. If handled positively, our failures may be the pivoting point ahead of tomorrow's success.

Secondly, seek divine direction. Omniscience is an attribute, possessed only by the Almighty God. Never be afraid to enquire of the Almighty regarding his purpose for your life. Our humanity limits our vision, but we have an opportunity to come boldly before the Throne of Grace and receive clarity as the Almighty gives us the desires of our hearts.

Thirdly, search diligently for the purpose behind the pain and as my former CEO would say, the gift in the experience. Don't be offended when people imply that you are allowed to suffer so that you could help others to find an easier way out. Remember that the only thing potentially worse than some of the pains we suffered is the thought of those experiences being in vain. No pain should be wasted. Every pain is attached to purpose.

Resources

Instagram: @predestined.women.empowerment

Facebook: @PredestinedforWomen

Website: https://fem.events

CHAPTER 31

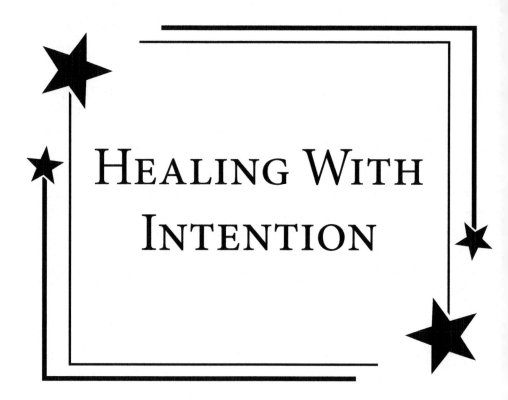

HEALING WITH INTENTION

BY: **DR. PEARNEL BELL**

Dr. Pearnel Bell

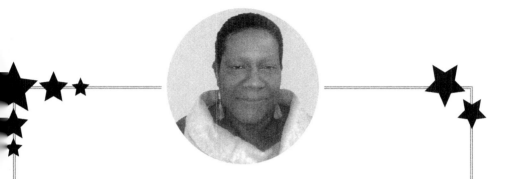

Dr. Pearnel Bell is a Clinical Psychologist and a Human Resource Consultant, with combined experience of over twenty-two years. These skills sets have been an asset as she skillfully navigates between workplace empowerment and helping individuals and groups recover from life's challenges. She has over the past twenty years worked closely with executives helping them develop leadership qualities and management skills, and assisting employees in progressing their careers by building skills for the next-level job position. She conducts psychological and psychometric tests, evaluating the performance of executives and staff helping them to identify strengths and how to maximize them while working on improving weaknesses. She has a Ph.D. in Psychology, a master's degree in Human Resource Management, and Post Graduate Certificate in Clinical Psychology from Walden University. She is currently a professor at Yorkville University and City University in Canada where she lectures in Ethics and Legal Issues, Human Development and Diversity and Culture. She is the author of eight books. Six therapeutic books for children, A Teachers Guide to Understanding Mental Disorders in Children and a therapeutic book for poetry therapy. Dr. Bell is an international speaker and has presented at many conferences in the USA and Canada. She had the awesome pleasure of supporting the team of co-authors in this volume.

HEALING WITH INTENTION

We all, at sometime in our lives, experience challenges. I remember years ago when I was completing my first degree, I had an encounter with an instructor who lost six months of my journal entries which was a requirement for her course. I was totally devastated and felt like I was spiralling into depression. One morning after many weeks, I had an awakening: Was I going to continue to drown in self-pity resulting in failing my course and failing the entire programme? I got up at that moment and began to write in my journal once again with renewed vigour. I had discovered at that moment that life is difficult. I also discovered that writing is therapy and has tremendous healing power.

Many years after I continued life's journey, I had come to realize that life is full of challenges. I almost lost my 16-year-old daughter in death, experienced a divorce, and it was writing my narrative that was the most healing. I wrote my first book, Words Once Unspoken: Poetry Inspired by Friendship. I totally embraced Ma Angelou's words when she wrote "There is no greater agony than bearing an untold story inside you."

I am now a therapist who has so forcefully learned that we must tell our stories, because untold stories manifest themselves in psychopathology, such as depression and anxiety. I have fully embraced the fundamentals of writing the narrative of our story because that is healing.

How do we then heal from authoring our story? The untold story becomes a rumination that is going nowhere. We become burdened in pain and agony for the rest of our lives as the story of our loss becomes the rest of our lives. Forgetting that there was a past and there is yet a future, we become stuck; life is no longer worth living. Our inner thoughts become our inner critic--that voice that rings too loud and never shuts up, it is our death sentence, if you may. We are alive, walking, breathing yet dead to our hopes, dreams, and future accomplishments, all gone because our perspective has become warped.

In my current practice I help clients to understand that healing can come from re-storying and changing the narrative. Narrative therapy is a powerful tool that helps clients examine their stories from a rational and empowering stance. It begins with us examining the dominant discourse. The current story we are telling ourselves gets mired into negativity. Its manifestation only seeks to make us feel lost in a world that we feel is always against us, hurling one terrible thing after another. This is it: I am alive but dead. People are around me, but I am lonely. I have good days, but they do not count, they are like flickers of the wick of a candle and I know no joy.

Narrative therapy helps us to see that both situations we experience are true, but we have internalised the problem and made it our own. It defines who we are–just a person swallowed up by loss and grief., Yes that is who we are, as we continue to internalise and become what we believe the loss has given us.

Re-storying and rewriting the narrative show us that we can externalise the problem. We can begin the process of taking the loss outside of ourselves and name it, yes name the problem, give it a name. My loss could be named, Pam, Albert, Crosses, Grief, Pain or Hurt. We should be aware that whatever name we choose to give our loss is entirely up to us. Doing this helps us to see what we are dealing with and helps invariably to begin the separation process–separating from the problem. It is now outside of ourselves, and we can now begin to view the problem in the third person as if there is a third person in the room. It can be seen as a thing or person that was exerting control over you. In naming the problem you now examine how "Pam" has been impacting you. How do you want to deal with the impact of "Pam"? The next step would be to look for ways to disempower it.

As we go through our loss, we tend to only see ourselves being engulfed in the pain of the loss; but the truth is as we navigate life through our pain there are unique outcomes that have been happening to us, but we were not paying attention to them because of the pain of our loss. In our narrative, we want to ask and answer the question: Since I have been experiencing my loss, what are the unique outcomes? What happened to me when I was not focused on the loss? How have I disempowered the grief? Invariably there are unique outcomes that we have experienced or benefitted from as a result of our loss. This is the time to take note of them and embrace those unique exceptions as an indication that healing can come from being engulfed in pain and hurt.

As you examine these exceptions to the pain and hurt, also look at how this loss is helping to form your identity: How am I now describing myself because of my loss? What is it that I want? Is my current situation where I want to be? If not, what are my next steps? Writing the narrative helps one to challenge the dominant, usually negative discourse that prevents one from engaging in life in a meaningful way. It helps those experiencing loss to restory –looking at the loss through different lenses, develop alternative stories. It certainly helps to challenge dysfunctional and unhealthy beliefs and assumptions. It opens the way for individuals to see the alternative, and to see that loss does not have to be prolonged but there can certainly be new beginnings to a life worth living.

As we rewrite our stories from loss to hope to new possibilities, it is important that we go through grief in a healthy way. As we face loss there are some key points from Positive Psychology to remember:. All our lived experiences are here to teach us about the human condition. This means we should embrace the notion of self-compassion. Self-compassion is crucial to our healing. We normally are compassionate to others in their times of grief but tend to be self-critical when we are experiencing a loss. The idea of self-compassion examines three key cornerstone,. namely, self-kindness vs. self-judgement, common humanity vs. isolation, and mindfulness vs. overidentification.

Let us examine each one on its own merit: We need to show ourselves kindness in times of loss rather than take on the stance of being self-judging. This is the time to speak to ourselves as we would to a friend who is having a similar experience. What would we say to such a friend? We would fill them with encouraging and empowering thoughts, comfort coupled with words of wisdom. Would we be judgmental? No way! Our empathetic skills would chime in, and we would end up providing guidance full of wisdom and kindness. Self-compassion is saying do the same for yourself as you know how. Who knows us better than ourselves and knows what our needs are?. Who better to provide such kindness and comfort but ourselves?. We should make kindness toward self an everyday occurrence.

We also must practise, as part of self-compassion, an understanding of common humanity vs. isolation. Nothing that has ever happened to us is certainly unique to us, it is part of the human condition, we are not in isolation with what we are facing, it is all part of the human experience. We should avoid asking 'why me'? because inherent in that question is why not someone else. It is prudent to ask what lessons am I learning about myself, life, the world, and others? Remembering that we are never alone, every circumstance we face is part of our common humanity.

Practise mindfulness vs. overidentification. Mindfulness is staying in the present moment to observe and accept thoughts, feelings as they come. It is the ability to be non-judgmental but more accepting and open to what is happening in the here and now. Mindfulness allows us not to over identify with the problem but accept rather than deny them. This helps us to embrace self-compassion and help with our acknowledgment of our current circumstances.

Another powerful technique for dealing with loss and grief comes from energy psychology. A technique called Emotional Freedom Technique or Tapping. Tapping is a technique that is based on the premise that our meridian points in the body are the areas that hold our emotional upsets resulting in the retention of hurt and pain in the body. Tapping on these areas of the body releases the negative emotions that are impacting the person. The main meridian points are named the karate chop, the eyebrow, side of the eye, under the eye, under the nose, on the chin, under the arm and on top of the head. The person starts with a set up statement relevant to the issues affecting them while validating and accepting their situation and themselves. The person begins with tapping and using the set-up statement "I release all my grief stress now. The person continues tapping that they want to overcome this grief. The person uses positive antidotes to grief such as I want more love, wisdom, more logic, power, etc. while tapping and asking for more of the positive energy the person wants.

In my mind one of the most fundamental lessons we learned when we experience loss and are in grief is to acknowledge that what we are going through is not unique to us but is part of the inheritance of what common humanity faces. We do not hide away from grieving and acknowledging the pain of the loss. What we do is accept and go through the process of grief. The stories of grief and loss are many; and many have also worked through their grief to develop hope and courage to tell their stories, to teach life lessons that we can move from scars to stars with intentional healing.

INTENTIONAL HEALING: FROM SCARS TO STARS

CHAPTER 32

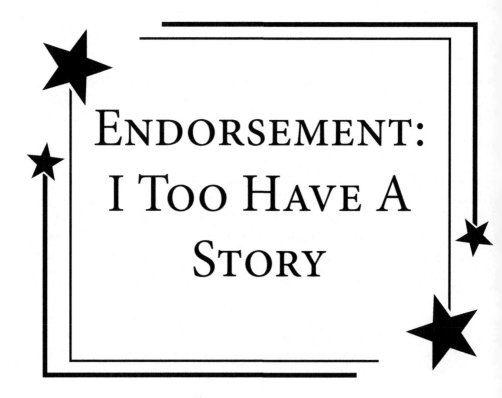

ENDORSEMENT: I TOO HAVE A STORY

BY: **DR. ERNIE E. R. WRIGHT JR.**

DR. ERNIE E. R. WRIGHT JR.

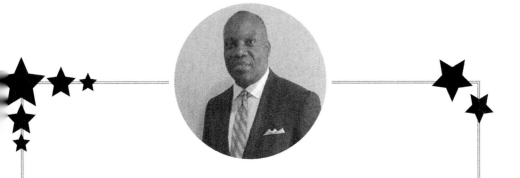

Ernie Wright was born on the breathtakingly beautiful Island of Jamaica. He started playing the piano at the age of six. Ernie had the distinct privilege of Performing on National television in Jamaica while a teenager. He attended Northern Caribbean University where he received a BA in Theology. He graduated from Andrews University with a MA in Religion and received an Honorary Doctorate of Divinity from Agape College. He studied music at Trinity College and The Royal School of Music. Ernie sang with the Rutgers University choir while on tour in Scotland. He conducted many choirs and led many singing groups both in Jamaica and the United States. He taught music in College and also privately. He plays the piano/keyboard and organ and emcees on special occasions. As an ordained SDA minister, he currently serves as the Senior Pastor of Redemption Praise Temple in Queens, New York. Ernie has been married to Cheryl née Ming for over 40 years. Together they have two adult children Garry and Kimberly. He is also the proud grandfather of Jelani and Charli. His favorite saying is "If God brings you to it He will take you through it."

ENDORSEMENT:
I TOO HAVE A STORY

I may not have the scientific language to define or interpret Intentional Healing from Scars to Stars. However, when I think of intentional healing, it is my expressed understanding that the individual has to take deliberate steps towards healing. 'Scars to stars' connote movement from one place to another, from one state of mind to another, and from one situation to another. Basically, it's the transformation of a negative thing or experience to something positive. Scars generally suggest that you've been battered or bruised, while stars suggest upward mobility. A star, whether in Hollywood or the Kingdom of God, is a visible proliferation of light and beauty that is suggestive of success and accomplishment while promising a more hopeful future.

I have many scars, but the most profound is my wife's battle with breast cancer and its impact. Though she has remained meaningfully engaged, she hasn't been formally employed for quite some time. As a nurse who has served as a nurse manager in a large hospital, Cheryl has always committed to living a healthy lifestyle. Exercising together was one of our favorite pastimes. Now on her better days, she can barely manage simple power walks and jogs. So, as her supportive husband, I've responded to every life-changing experience though she struggled to remain my jovial, spontaneous, optimistic, and cheerful love. I miss my goal-oriented, purpose-driven, creative, sassy servant leader who had such grace, elegance, and poise as a professional. Even though those desirable things are missed, my greatest desire is for her to be healthy again. I've watched her most pleasurable and effortless activities such as gardening and decorating become tedious chores as she is often tired. This new normal is one I am still grappling to accept and like the co-authors, I do feel down at times.

Before things changed, life was a little freer and easier. But then there are persons, some of whom are featured i this anthology, like Dr. Grace, my sister Patrice, Ray, and Carmen, who help me not just to pass the day, but to enjoy one day at a time. The good days become accumulative. I also benefit from the valuable support of the Redemption Praise Temple family, my biological family, and extended friends. I also have learnt to name and publicly acknowledge my pain without feeling bad. I acknowledge that I have had scars and navigate them everyday by engaging in activities that help me to focus on some pleasantries of life. I also do a lot of self-care and remain focused on supporting my members and building my ministry in my pastoral capacity. I keep so busy that, even though my wife and I were the first to have been invited to be a part of this book programme, we missed the opportunity of having our story in this volume.

This anthology is not just a compilation of stories. It's the end result of a life-transforming process. Grieving with Dr. Grace has helped us to realise how one reacts to pain and loss. Grief is a natural response to pain. During the writing process, I was able to appreciate that I've grieved about things other than my father's death and have failed to acknowledge many other things for which I have been or should have been grieving. I really applaud the work that Dr. Grace has done in supporting these authors to be able to retell and not relive their stories and have the courage to publish for the benefit of others. My wife and I, and members of our congregation, are proud benefactors of her grief coaching and support. I have watched some of these authors navigate their scars and transition from brokenness to wholeness, from pain to purpose, and now leave glitter on the lives of others. I know these stories will empower many as she continues to traverse the globe offering support to wounded hearts.

I might be repeating what I said earlier, but it is always good to write things down so your legacy can be memorialized and outlive you. My wife Cheryl and I will have our story in Volume II and hope that if you too missed Volume I, you will join us. I salute each author. I am particularly encouraged by the stories of Dawn and Stacia, who themselves have shared snippets about breast cancer, and Jodine, who has been navigating her autoimmune challenges.

I fully endorse this as a masterful piece of work adding much value to the literature, stories of healing, courage, strength, and hope.

- Dr. Ernie E. R. Wright Jr.

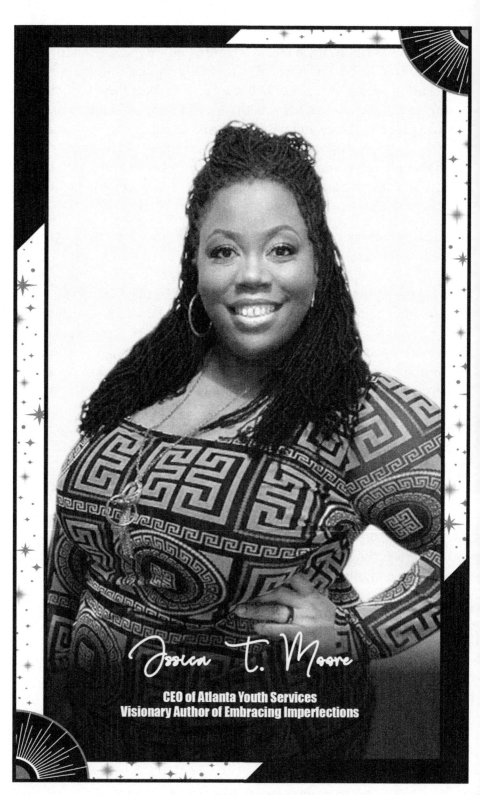

Jessica T. Moore

CEO of Atlanta Youth Services
Visionary Author of Embracing Imperfections

AFTERWORD

Dr. Grace A. Kelly has led a team of people to write a must-read primer book on healing. As one of my co-authors who has published stories in two of my books. Dr. Grace showed tremendous potential; Because of her persistence, I welcomed her to be a part of Volumes II and III. She went on to join my program as a visionary author and I am proud of her for being courageous in her pursuit to help others to own their stories.

It is a joy for me to see that despite her challenges with being dyslexic, she managed to navigate her scars to be shining as one of my star visionary authors. You see, I have to work through my own scars of grief, having lost my mother at a young age and becoming a teen mom. With these scars, I do identify with many of the co-authors and with Dr. Grace who has defied the odds. Her being able to lead 31 people from across the globe, with varied scars from physical ailments, death, dying and social ills, is in itself a sign of an overcomer who herself has embraced her imperfections, stuck with the program, and got results.

Those familiar with my message know that I love the concept of standing on your story and not in it. As a visionary author of my own book series, Embracing Imperfections, I love how this book was beautifully put together. Intentional Healing from Scars to Stars is a delightful read filled with inspirational stories for those of us who want to enjoy a good read while learning how to heal intentionally and navigate our scars to become stars.

- Jessica T. Moore

Conclusion By
Dr. Grace A. Kelly

My effort in this anthology, Intentional Healing: From Scars to Stars, has been to articulate an understanding that everyone, at some point in his/her life, will encounter situations that will cause them pain. As one who has been through so much pain, too numerous to narrate, I have vowed that, as long as I can help or direct someone to the help they deserve, they should not have to suffer and navigate their grief alone. Regardless of age, sex, education, socio-economic, or socio-political status, those painful encounters may inevitably lead to scars, some of which can be debilitating and life-altering.

As we traverse this journey called life, many of us can attest to the agonizing experiences that have scarred us. If having read this book, you realize that scars are a common thread amongst many of us and you see that it is possible to embark on your healing journey where your scars can be transformed into stars, then our objective would have been met to allow you, the reader, to know that healing is possible.

I am supposing that after having read this book, you recognize that in order for true healing to take place, you have to be intentional about changing your perceptions and your actual circumstances. In that case, you are ready to start your healing journey and yet another objective would have been met.

The authored stories have been deliberately compiled to highlight the various methods by which these authors were able to transform their scars into stars by altering their behaviors and thought processes which is crucial to healing hurting hearts. Collectively, the contributing authors had one goal in mind and that was to speak their truth to inspire others to break the silence, end the cycle of abuse, and overcome the crippling effects of their scars. They wanted you to recognize that you are not alone and you have the God-given power to allow your pain to fuel your passion for liberation, transform your pain into purpose, and mobilize your dreams to be the best version of yourself.

To experience freedom from the shackles and scars of guilt, shame, grief, abuse, and rejection, it takes commitment to yourself and to the processes outlined in this book, to help you navigate the arduous but satisfying journey of healing, which leads to the transformation of scars to shining stars. If this was realized, then we can be satisfied that God has used us to be conduits of His blessings to you. My absolute pleasure serving you and to God be the glory.

Allow me to end with this quote from one of my favourite authors:

It will not be long until we see Him in whom our hopes of eternal life are centered. And in His presence, all the trials and sufferings of this life will be as nothingness.... Look up, look up, and let your faith continually increase. Let this faith guide you along the narrow path that leads through the gates of the city of God into the great beyond, the wide, unbounded future of glory that is for the redeemed. White, E. G. Our Father Cares p.102

ABOUT THE VISIONARY AUTHOR
DR. GRACE A. KELLY

Dr. Grace A. Kelly is an Associate Professor and Administrator at Northern Caribbean University and a Past President of the Jamaica Association of Guidance Counsellors in Education (JAGCE). Her philanthropic commitments have led to her service as Volunteer Chaplain with the Jamaica Constabulary Force, Board Member with the Manchester Peace Coalition, The Salvation Army Windsor Lodge Children's Home, a Member of the Manchester Chamber of Commerce, Manchester Parish Development Committee, and other areas of service.

Dr. Grace Kelly has contributed significantly to research in the areas of Children's Advocacy; At-Risk Youth; Grief Recovery, Death, Dying and Bereavement; Comprehensive Guidance Counselling; and Restorative Justice in Schools. She is a passionate Community Development Worker, who has worked with a number of Churches and a wide range of local and international Governmental and Non-Governmental Community-Based organizations to develop, implement, and positively impact community and nation-building efforts.

Dr. Kelly has received numerous awards for her philanthropy endeavors, the most recent being the 2019 Governor General's Achievement Award for the parish of Manchester. As a counsellor and educator, Dr. Kelly has positively impacted the lives of many. She is a Grief and Bereavement Therapist-Coach and a Crisis Interventionist and Restorative Justice practitioner. She is the Host of the online programme, Let's Talk Life and Legacy: A Moment with Dr. Grace.

A four-time Amazon Best-Selling Author, and Author of the book Grieve If You Must: A 21-day Plan for Grieving, Healing, and Restoration, Dr. Kelly's philosophy is that "grieving is to pain, as breathing is to life." Through her influence, these co-authors have been inspired to use their own painful yet overcoming experiences with grief to positively impact the lives of others, by retelling, but not reliving their stories.

There are free resources and access to a suite of services available for you. Visit us at
www.theolivebranchgloballlc.com.

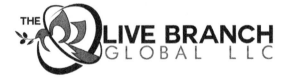

Printed in Great Britain
by Amazon

10792497R00174